Food Allergy

FOOD ALLERGY

Second Edition

Frederic Speer, M.D.

Director, Speer Allergy Clinic, Shawnee Mission, Kansas;
  Clinical Professor of Pediatrics, University of Kansas,
  Kansas City, Kansas.

WITHDRAWN

John Wright • PSG Inc
Boston   Bristol   London
1983

To my wife, Jeannette Hybskmann Speer, and to our children, Susan, Mary, Julia, Martha, Stuart, Clara, Ruth, Helen, and Mark, with all my affection and appreciation. In one way or another all have been closely involved in my long interest in foods and food allergy.

Library of Congress Cataloging in Publication Data

Speer, Frederic.
    Food allergy.

    Bibliography: p.
    Includes index.
    1. Food allergy. I. Title. [DNLM: 1. Food
hypersensitivity. WD 310 S742f]
RC596.S68 1983   616.9'75   82-17664
ISBN 0-7236-7016-1

Published simultaneously by:
John Wright • PSG Inc, 545 Great Road, Littleton,
Massachusetts 01460 U.S.A.
John Wright & Sons, Ltd., 823–825 Bath Road,
Bristol BS4 5NU, England

First Edition © *1978*
Second Printing 1979

Second Edition © *1983*

Printed in Great Britain
Bound in the United States of America

International Standard Book Number 0-7236-7016-1

Library of Congress Catalog Card Number: 82-17664

CONTENTS

PREFACE TO FIRST EDITION

Defined narrowly, the term allergy is limited to illness caused by a demonstrable antigen/antibody reaction. An excellent example is ragweed hay fever. But so narrow a definition falls short. Many obvious allergic reactions occur in which there is no objective evidence whatever of an immunologic reaction. This is the rule in drug allergy; in only an occasional case can the offending drug be identified immunologically.

Another class of allergens seldom identifiable by immunologic methods is foods. As a result, food allergy is widely overlooked, and its victims may not even be recognized as allergic patients. Their complaints, which are often diffuse and poorly defined, are written off as idiopathic, psychosomatic, or imaginary. Such people often must endure, in addition to the distress caused by food allergy, both the indignity of being labeled neurotic and the frustration of not having the cause of their illness recognized.

This tendency to confuse allergy with emotional illness is not as modern as might be supposed. In 1865 the following report was published of two unhappy mothers of babies who would now be immediately recognized as allergic:

> A poor woman, a neighbor of mine, was confined in the upper story of her house; her husband was dying in the room below. We might ask: Could the child escape under such circumstances? No: it was covered a few days after its birth with eczema. Within the last week a young woman brought in her babe to me covered with eczema from head to foot. The colloquy which took place between myself and the parent was as follows: "How old is your child?" "Four months." "How long has he had the eruption?" "Since he was three weeks old." "What occurred immediately before the appearance of the disease in your child to cause you annoyance?" "I was vexed by my servant." "And what since?" "I have been vexed to see my poor child in this miserable state."[213]

Sad to say, well over a century later we cannot hold that this cavalier "psychosomatic" approach is a thing of the past. Scarcely a day passes that the allergist does not hear a patient say something like, "I have been told it's my nerves." Many patients are on tranquilizers, and some have been subjected to group therapy or some other method designed to relieve neurotic and hysterical ills.

The management of food allergy begins with identification of the responsible allergens. This is the *first* major emphasis of this book. Since objective tests are of little more than marginal value, successful detection must depend on a thorough knowledge of foods (the cause) and clinical manifestations (the effect). Both foods and manifestations will therefore receive extended attention.

After food allergens are identified and eliminated, the next step is to provide the patient with a diet that is at once allergen-free, acceptable, and nourishing. This is the *second* major emphasis of the book.

Working out the problems of a patient with food allergy is always challenging and may be difficult. But the physician who takes these problems seriously will find that no clinical experience is more rewarding and that no patient is more grateful.

Frederic Speer, M.D.

PREFACE TO SECOND EDITION

For many years the field of food allergy has suffered from neglect. It is often held to be unimportant, unscientific, even nonexistent. In recent years this trend has been reversed, and in the four years since the first edition of this book was published, much new and valuable clinical material has appeared. This material has been used to enrich and expand this edition. Revision has been especially extensive in the following chapters:

Chapter 2. Confusion is often caused by considering all adverse reactions to foods as allergic reactions. Included in this revised chapter is new material on commonly overlooked food items that may cause toxic reactions.

Chapter 4. Added to the classification of food allergens included in the first edition, already the most complete in print, are a number of additional items. Another new feature of this chapter is a group of drawings showing the morphological similarities of biologically related plant foods. They make more vivid these important relationships and make cross-reactivity more easily understood.

Chapter 5. This chapter, the most important and detailed of all, is devoted to an expanded discussion of the foods themselves. A new feature is a table listing the names of common foods in English, French, Spanish, Italian, and German. This is eminently practical—in the management of food allergy there must be no language barrier between physician and patient.

Chapter 9. In adults and older children, food allergy is always a source of suffering and disability, but in infants it can be extremely dangerous. In this revised chapter is reflected the increasing interest being paid by pediatricians to this important subject.

Frederic Speer, M.D.

ACKNOWLEDGMENTS

As with my other books and papers, my wife, Jeannette Hybskmann Speer, has been of irreplaceable help in matters of content and style. In this book she has made the further contribution of writing the major part of Chapter 8. She has tried all of the recipes listed in the chapter and found them practical and, for the most part, easy to prepare. And I have found the results to be delicious.

My special thanks to W. H. Freeman and Company for permission to reproduce the list of additives in Table 5-2.

My thanks go also to the following authors and publishers for permission to reproduce their valuable material: HJ Roberts, American Medical Association; PL White, American Medical Association; V Herbert, American Medical Association and Florida Medical Association; WJ Darby, Florida Medical Association; T Furia, CRC Press.

FS

1 • INTRODUCTION

Food allergy is a form of immediate hypersensitivity, or atopy, closely related to inhalant allergy. According to the classification of Coombs and Gell, it falls under the heading of the type I, or anaphylactic, reaction.* Here I have used four terms: allergy, hypersensitivity, atopy, and anaphylactic. Throughout the book I will generally use the term *allergy*. *Hypersensitivity,* a somewhat cumbersome synonym for allergy, serves no purpose and will be avoided. *Atopy,* a more precise term, will be used only when precision is called for. *Anaphylactic* and its parent word *anaphylaxis* are, in the United States and Canada at least, reserved for systemic reactions resembling the anaphylactic shock of experimental animals.

Although the two are grouped together as immediate reactions, food allergy and inhalant allergy are not identical. It is true that they cause similar manifestations and affect the same type of patient. But the differences are real, and only when this is realized is proper management of food allergy possible. These differences may be summarized as follows:

1. Food allergy tends to cause a wide variety of manifestations, often constituting a systemic disturbance. Inhalant allergy tends to be limited in scope, affecting principally (but not exclusively) the respiratory tract.
2. Food allergy usually causes gastrointestinal disturbances. Inhalant allergy seldom does.
3. Food allergy often begins in early childhood and may be present at birth. Inhalant allergy is unusual under the age of two years and rare under the age of one year.
4. Except in severe cases (and not always then), food sensitization is seldom revealed by skin tests or other objective methods. These procedures are usually accurate in inhalant allergy.
5. Reactions to foods are usually delayed for several hours and last for several days. Reactions to inhalants tend to come on within minutes and if exposure is not continued, to disappear in an hour or so.

---

*Coombs RRA, Gell PGH: Classification of allergic reactions responsible for clinical hypersensitivity and diseases. In Coombs RRA, Gell PGH eds: *Clinical Aspects of Immunology,* 2nd ed. Philadelphia, FA Davis, 1968, p 575.

6. Hyposensitization, a common method of treating inhalant allergy, is not effective in food allergy.
7. In almost every case, detection of food allergens depends on clinical methods, chiefly elimination and challenge.

Two of the differences between food allergy and inhalant allergy are to be expected. We could expect foods to cause disturbances in the gastrointestinal tract, the first and heaviest point of contact. And because food allergens enter the system while inhalants stay mostly on or near the surface, we could expect foods to cause a constitutional disturbance. Rowe and other pioneer observers thought that the liver might be where food allergens are active.[157] It is possible that mediators are released there to be dispersed throughout the body. This might also account for the fact that reactions to foods are both slow to appear and slow to disappear.

Three other questions remain unanswered. We do not know why food allergy is so often present at birth, why hyposensitization is ineffective, or why skin tests and other objective tests are usually negative. The presence of food allergy at birth has been attributed to intrauterine sensitization. This is a possibility, but it does not explain why milk allergy, the most common food sensitivity, is often present at birth in infants born of mothers who never take milk in any form. We commonly see this in whole families. We cannot say why hyposensitization is ineffective in food allergy nor even make an educated guess—as far as that goes, we do not know why it *is* effective in inhalant allergy. The failure of such tests as the radioallergosorbent test, skin tests, and histamine release indicates that the nature of food allergy is ordinarily radically different from the more familiar and better understood inhalant allergy. This is discussed later in this chapter under the heading of Mechanism of Food Allergy.

HISTORY OF FOOD ALLERGY

The intolerance to foods which we now call allergy has been recognized for centuries. Since these reactions are sometimes violent, our remote ancestors must have known that what we call anaphylactic shock could be brought on by ordinarily wholesome foods. Undoubtedly such crises were generally considered to represent punishment of the gods, but as early as the first century B.C. Lucretius had the insight to see that intolerance is an individual peculiarity entirely unrelated to the nature of the food. His comment on the problem has been widely quoted: *Quod ali cibus est aliis fuat acre venenum* (What is food to one may be fierce poison to others). In the early seventeenth century Beaumont and Fletcher echoed the same thought: "What's one man's poison, signor, is another's meat and drink."

Samuel Pepys made this entry in his diary on September 5, 1664:

> "Came W. Bowyer and dined with us; but strange to see how he could not endure onyons in sauce to lamb, but was overcome by the sight of it so was forced to make his dinner from an egg or two."[3]

It was not until the nineteenth century that physicians began to pay serious attention to what was then called food idiosyncrasy. One of the early reports on the role of foods in asthma appeared in the 1840–41 issue of *Lancet.* It is worthy of note that the author, H. A. Roods, believed asthma attacks to be mediated through the vagus (pneumogastric) nerve, a view that is now standard.

> In the case of a gentleman who has been for many years subject to attacks of spasmodic asthma of a very severe character, and for whom I have long been in the habit of prescribing, the attack has invariably appeared to have been the result of, and occasioned by, errors in diet; if he partook freely either of veal, salted meat, pastry or various other edibles, an embarrassment of the respiratory functions, to a greater or less degree, usually supervened about half an hour or an hour afterwards; and although many slight attacks of this description passed off quickly, yet they frequently increased in intensity, and terminated in extremely violent paroxysms of spasmodic asthma. The inference drawn from these facts is, that the paroxysms alluded to resulted from a morbid impression made on the gastric branches of the pneumo-gastric nerve, which impairment was conveyed through the trunk and pulmonary branches of this nerve to the mucous membrane of the air passages, where it produced some functional derangement, the effects of which were the phenomena constituting the malady in question.[156]

In 1855 there appeared a detailed account of a man whose asthma and constitutional symptoms were caused by wheat. This report is remarkable not only for being one of the pioneer observations of what is now called food allergy, but also because the author brings out four points now known to be important: 1) food allergy tends to cause a tremendous increase in mucous secretions; 2) in severe cases the odor of the offending food may cause symptoms; 3) food allergy may begin immediately after birth, even at the first feeding; and 4) many people ignore the patient's insistence that he cannot eat a given food, "not believing in his infirmity."

4

This report was presented by Overton (otherwise unidentified) and appeared in the *Southern Journal of Medical and Physical Sciences,* Vol. 3, 1855.

> The patient was throughout life, from his cradle to his grave, the victim of what is possibly a unique idiosyncrasy of constitution. In his own words he declared: "Of two equal parts of tartar and wheat flour...I would rather swallow the tartar than the wheat flour." If he ate flour in any form or however combined, in the smallest quantity, in two minutes or less he would have painful itching over the whole body, accompanied by severe colic and tormina in the bowels, great sickness in the stomach, and continued vomiting, which he declared was ten times as distressing as the symptoms caused by the ingestion of tartar emetic. In about ten minutes after eating the flour the itching would be greatly intensified, especially about the head, face, and eyes, but tormenting all parts of the body, and not to be appeased. These symptoms continued for two days with intolerable violence, and only declined on the third day and ceased on the tenth. In the convalescence, the lungs were affected, he coughed, and in expectoration raised great quantities of phlegm, and really resembled a phthisical patient. At this time he was confined to his room with great weakness, similar to that of a person recovering from an asthmatic attack. The mere smell of wheat produced distressing symptoms in a minor degree, and for this reason he could not, without suffering, go into a mill or house where the smallest quantity of wheat flour was kept. His condition was the same from the earliest times, and he was laid out for dead when an infant at the breast, after being fed with "pap" thickened with wheat flour....One of his female neighbors, not believing in his infirmity, but considering it only a whim, put a small quantity of flour in the soup which she gave him to eat at her table, stating that it contained no flour, and as a consequence of the deception he was bedridden for ten days with his usual symptoms.[77]

From these two case reports, both appearing well over a century ago, it is obvious that food allergy, whatever it is called, has long been recognized.

At the close of the nineteenth century and during the opening years of the twentieth a number of observers began to correlate clinical experience with laboratory findings to show that what had been called idiosyncrasy was an immunologic phenomenon. It is interesting that as early as 1885 Bulkley had pointed out that urticaria, eczema, and asthma had a common origin.[26] He credited Sir Andrew Clark with suggesting this five years previously. Bulkley made the significant comment that these diseases "may result from some altered condition of the blood."

The role of "some altered condition of the blood" in disease was discovered independently by Charles Richet and Paul Portier in 1902 and by Clemens von Pirquet in 1906. Richet introduced the term *anaphylaxis* and von Pirquet, *allergy*. There is evidence that their observations had been anticipated by François Magendie in 1839, and, as Unger and Harris point out, the credit for first working with allergy should be shared by Charles Blackley, Morrill Wyman, Maurice Arthus, Theobald Smith, Simon Flexner, Bela Schick, and others.[148]

The physicians of the early years of the twentieth century had a problem—they hardly knew what to make of the new discoveries which indicated that the old idiosyncrasy was the new allergy or, perhaps, anaphylaxis. Early confidence that food allergens could be detected easily by skin tests raised hopes that foods could be implicated in all sorts of obscure diseases. When it was seen that many a negative test concealed valid sensitivity, interest in food allergy went into a decline from which it has never fully recovered. It need not have done so if this early (1917) caution of Talbot had been taken seriously: "Up-to-date the writer has not been able to establish any connection between these diseases and foods by means of skin tests, and it is possible that some other method of diagnosis would have to be devised."[190]

Credit for keeping interest in food allergy alive can go to many clinicians but especially to Albert H. Rowe of California. He refused to be bound by the skin test or any other laboratory procedure and stoutly maintained through his long career that food allergy, no matter how little evidence of its existence comes from research, is common, important, and tragically overlooked. Our modern approach to the detection of food allergens rests on his famous elimination diets.[157]

MECHANISM OF FOOD ALLERGY

When food allergy is severe, that is, when a small amount of allergen provokes an immediate and obvious reaction, it resembles inhalant allergy. Under these conditions objective methods of identification of antibody may be positive. When such potent allergens as peanut, egg, and fish behave in this way, skin tests, RAST, and other methods of demonstrating an antigen-antibody reaction are often positive. In fact, the passive transfer test of Prausnitz and Küstner was first demonstrated with serum containing antibody against fish.

But most cases of food allergy are much more subtle than this, seldom revealing objective evidence of an immunologic reaction other than the clinical manifestations. In an attempt to divorce food allergy from inhalant allergy, Coca in 1953 suggested the name "familial, non-reaginic food allergy."[32]

Although what we know about food allergy seldom fits in with what we know about classic inhalant atopy, our hope of better understanding rests on continued study of the atopic reaction. The following is a brief review.

Atopy

Atopy is a variation or exaggeration of a normal humoral response in man. Early investigators recognized that something in serum, presumably an antibody, was responsible for its manifestations. It was given the name of *reagin* by Coca. Thanks to the brilliant researches of Ishizaka and Ishizaka, reagin is now known to be an immunoglobulin, called IgE, normally present in minute amounts in human serum.[98] It is possible that some immunoglobulin G (IgG) has reaginic properties when causing urticaria, angioedema, and certain other reactions. In these cases it may act by initiating an immune complex disorder rather than an atopic reaction.

Most antibody is produced by plasma cells, which are found in high concentration in the respiratory and gastrointestinal tracts. It has a strong affinity for mast cells in tissue and basophils in the blood. The atopic reaction is initiated when two IgE molecules attached to the cell are bridged by antigen. This triggers a chain of enzyme reactions with the release of histamine and other vasocative factors, especially "slow reacting substance of anaphylaxis" (SRSA). Histamine causes vasodilatation and increased capillary permeability, which are responsible for the wheal-and-flare reaction of the skin test. SRSA, which causes prolonged contraction of smooth muscle, is thought to be the chief mediator of asthma.

IgE is measured either by weight or by units. The normal level by weight ranges from 1 ng* to 8,000 ng per ml. In atopic individuals the range is from about 25 ng to as high as 29,000 ng (29 µg) per ml.[10] Values are especially high in allergic eczema (atopic dermatitis). It is interesting that these patients tend to have unusually strong reactions to skin tests, many reactions being false positives.

One unit of IgE is that amount contained in 0.110284 mg of a freeze-dried pooled serum. It is equivalent to 2.35 ng of myeloma IgE or 2.42 ng of serum IgE. Myeloma IgE is not significantly different from serum IgE.

---

*One gram (g) equals 1,000 milligrams (mg) or 1,000,000 micrograms (µg) or 1,000,000,000 nanograms (ng).

In Vitro Detection of Food Sensitivity

The detection of sensitivity to foods remains pretty much what it was when allergy was first recognized, that is, elimination and challenge. In fact, the efficiency of all methods of detection, including skin tests and in vitro tests, is judged by how closely they correlate with clinical observation. There are, however, two reasons why in vitro tests should be taken seriously. One is that accurate objective tests are almost certain to be developed in the future. The other is that they teach us a great deal about the strange nature of atopy.

The Radioallergosorbent Test (RAST)   The RAST is undoubtedly the most ingenious laboratory method of detecting sensitivity and also the most accurate. It correlates closely with skin testing in inhalant sensitivity and in the severe type of immediate atopic reactions to foods. However, it is of little, if any, value in the common, delayed-onset type.

The RAST is a radioimmunoassay procedure designed to detect IgE antibody with specificity against a given allergen. It involves four steps: 1) the allergen is chemically bound to cellulose particles or discs; 2) this insoluble complex is added to the patient's serum, binding specific antibody and forming a new insoluble complex; 3) the new complex is washed, radioactive anti-IgE serum, labeled with either ^{125}I or ^{131}I, is added to it, and binding again occurs; and 4) the radioactivity of this complex is calculated, thereby measuring the amount of IgE specific for the allergen.[17]

Histamine release   The basis of this test is the release of histamine from the leukocytes of allergic and nonallergic individuals who have been sensitized by the serum of allergic patients. This occurs in the presence of allergen. Galant et al[71] and Dockhorn[53] have found that it has no practical application to food allergy.

Lymphocyte transformation   This test involves exposing cultured human lymphocytes to antigen. It has been considered more of a test of cellular immunity than atopy, but some observers believe it has some value in detecting IgE antibody. It is of no value in food allergy.

Rat Mast Cell Degranulation (RMCD) Test   Whether or not IgE will bind to the mast cells of rats or any other animals except primates is questionable, and most workers who have tried to bring this about have failed. There is therefore little hope that demonstration of degranulation in this test is meaningful. Even if it is, as Heiner has pointed out, the test is "tedious and requires compulsive detail."[88]

Skin window test   Eosinophils tend to appear when denuded

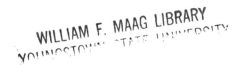

skin is exposed to allergens. The test is carried out by counting the eosinophils that accumulate under a coverslip used to occlude the denuded area. Galant et al found this test of no value in the detection of food allergens responsible for delayed-onset reactions and only 55% accurate in the immediate, severe type.[71]

Cytotoxic test An attempt has been made to identify food allergens by incubating leukocytes with allergen and the patient's serum. Positive tests have been described by changes in the morphology and mobility of leukocytes. Lieberman et al checked 15 patients with known food allergy, 10 patients with less well-defined allergic symptoms, and 20 controls. They found the procedure to be time consuming and completely inaccurate.[120] More recently a review of this technique by the American Academy of Allergy concluded: "There is no proof that leukocytoxic testing is effective for diagnosis of food or inhalant allergy."[2]

Immune Reactions in Food Allergy

Immune reactions are seldom demonstrable in the laboratory or by skin test, and Galant, Bullock, and Frick in their excellent review of the subject have discussed four theories to explain why.[71]

1. *The allergen may be a digestive product of the food rather than the food itself.* This commonly heard theory has little but speculation to support it. It would certainly not explain why the casein hydrolysate Nutramigen, described by the manufacturer as "predigested protein," is far less allergenic than casein itself. And there is no analogy here between food allergy and inhalant allergy since the intact proteins isolated from pollens are among our most potent allergens.

2. *The responsible antibody may not be IgE.* When we remember that it was only as late as 1966 that IgE was found to be the missing antibody in atopy, it is not unreasonable to speculate that some hitherto undiscovered reaginic antibody may account for most reactions to foods.

3. *A mediator other than histamine may be released in food allergy.* If we accept the possibility that a new immunoglobulin may be discovered, we can also accept the possibility that a new mediator may be discovered.

4. *The manifestations of most cases of food allergy are on a nonimmunologic basis.* With Galant and his co-workers, I totally reject this theory. It does not explain why food allergy causes typical allergic symptoms. It does not explain why food allergy is almost always accompanied by inhalant allergy. And it does not explain why many patients with inhalant allergy (to say nothing of drug allergy) have

negative skin tests. Pollen-sensitive patients almost always have positive skin tests, but many patients obviously allergic to molds and epidermals (especially dog hair) do not.

Whatever the ultimate explanation of the mechanism of food allergy, we can agree heartily with Galant and his co-workers when they say, "While these studies are in progress, the patient must be helped now. A careful history, in conjunction with the classic elimination diet and challenge, remain the most useful tools, at present, for the diagnosis of this form of food sensitivity."[71]

HEREDITY OF FOOD ALLERGY

One point on which all observers agree is that the tendency to develop an allergic disease is inherited. This tendency as it applies to food allergy was noticed long before allergy was thought of. In the 1800s Sir Morell Mackenzie received the following letter from "a distinguished litterateur":

> My daughter tells me that you are interested in the ill-effects which the eating of eggs has upon her, upon me, and upon my father before us. I believe my grandfather, as well as my father, could not eat eggs with impunity. As to my father himself, he is nearly eighty years old; he has not touched an egg since he was a young man; he can, therefore, give no precise or reliable account of the symptoms the eating of eggs produces in him. . . . As for me, the peculiarity was discovered when I was a spoonfed child. On several occasions it was noticed (that is my mother's account) that I felt ill without apparent cause; afterward it was recollected that a small part of a yolk of an egg had been given to me. Eclairissement came immediately after taking a single spoonful of egg. I fell into such an alarming state that the doctor was sent for. The effect seems to have been just the same that it produces upon my daughter now,—something that suggested brain-congestion and convulsions. From time to time, as a boy and young man, I have eaten an egg by way of trying it again, but always with the same result—a feeling that I had been poisoned; and yet all the while I liked eggs. Then I never touched them for years. Later I tried again, and I find the ill-effects are gradually wearing off. With my daughter it is different; she, I think, becomes more susceptible as time goes on, and the effect upon her is more violent than in my case at any time. Sometimes an egg has been put with coffee unknown to her, and she has been seen immediately afterward with her face alarmingly changed—eyes swollen and wild, the face crimson, the look of apoplexy. This is her own account: "An egg in any form causes within a few minutes great uneasiness and restlessness, the throat becomes contracted and painful, the face crimson, and the veins swollen. These symptoms have been so severe that serious consequences might follow." To this I may add that in her experience and my own, the newer the egg, the worse the consequences.[77]

10

This account indicates that food allergy as a family trait may include allergy to a given food. Here is a similar story supplied in 1919 by the pioneer allergist Guy LaRoche of Paris. He prefaces it by commenting, "The susceptibility of many members of the same family to eggs and milk is well known clinically."

> I have observed an unusual history of hereditary susceptibility to eggs. The most marked sensitization was in the great-grandfather. A cream or a meringue poisoned him. He had given up eating eggs since they produced vomiting, colic, and diarrhea. (Figure 1-1 shows a chart of the family history.)
>
> The intolerance of X remained legendary in this family. It was said that eggs poisoned him. His son had retained only a special susceptibility to cream and especially to meringue from the beaten white of eggs, either uncooked or partly cooked. To the daughters of Y, eggs were poisonous. Z had some definite attacks of vomiting after ingestion of cream, and she could tolerate only the yolks of eggs.[116]

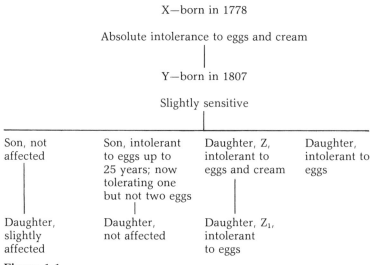

X—born in 1778

Absolute intolerance to eggs and cream

Y—born in 1807

Slightly sensitive

Son, not affected	Son, intolerant to eggs up to 25 years; now tolerating one but not two eggs	Daughter, Z, intolerant to eggs and cream	Daughter, intolerant to eggs
Daughter, slightly affected	Daughter, not affected	Daughter, Z_1, intolerant to eggs	

Figure 1-1

Families like the two cited here are seen by every allergist. But when it comes to explaining the mode of inheritance, there are many questions that cannot be answered at present. Cooke and Vanderveer believed that nearly three-quarters of children with a bilateral history of allergy eventually develop allergic disorders.[33] Bazaral et al have concluded that the atopic trait is a Mendelian dominant with partial penetrance.[13] Gerrard et al have confirmed what allergists have long suspected, that not only allergy itself but the tendency to develop a given disease is likely to be inherited. They found this to be true of asthma, hay fever, eczema, and perennial nasal allergy. It was not true, however, of urticaria.[72]

Whatever the explanation, allergy is obviously a family trait. This knowledge gives us the opportunity to take seriously not only the patient's complaints but those of his family. Many a new patient comments, "If you can help me, the rest of the family will probably be in."

INCIDENCE OF ALLERGY

When we consider how many disorders are caused by allergy and how many patients do not consult a physician about them, it is easy to see that we have no way of knowing how common they are. When surveys of populations have been made there has been considerable difference in the results. This undoubtedly depends on where the line is drawn as to what constitutes an allergic disease, the population surveyed, and the enthusiasm of those making the survey. Since most studies have been made by allergists, some bias toward calling a given disease an allergic disease is unavoidable. Table 1-1 summarizes these studies; it must be borne in mind that the table includes all sorts of allergy, not just food allergy.

Table 1-1
Incidence of Allergy

Observers	Population	Major Allergy	Minor Allergy
Appel et al[7]	Children	23.7%	
London[124]	Children	6.6%	32.0%
Arbeiter[8]	Adolescents	24.1%	
Jimenez[99]	College age	35.0%	20.0%
Vaughan[204]	All ages	10.0%	40–50%
Pipes[146]	All ages	13.0%	36.0%

2 • NONALLERGIC REACTIONS TO FOODS

When a study is being made of allergic reactions to foods, it must not be forgotten that every adverse reaction is not an allergic reaction. Some foods may be inherently toxic or are made so by contamination. And some patients have physical or metabolic defects that cause intolerance to certain foods.

TOXINS NATURALLY OCCURRING IN FOODS

The modern chemist, with his ultrasensitive analytical methods, has found that toxic substances are to be found in many, if not most, plant and animal foods. This is true whether foods are raw, smoked, salted, pickled, or otherwise modified, or whether they contain either deliberate or accidental additives. Fortunately these toxins are present in such minute amounts that they may be eaten without ill effects. This is especially true when the diet is diversified so that any given food is not eaten in excess. Some of the toxins found in common foods are discussed in Chapter 5. (See, as examples, ackee, additives, licorice, mushroom, nutmeg, poke, potato, rye.)

Vitamins

To an incredible extent, the American public has been persuaded that the average diet is lacking in vitamins. For this reason every drug store and food market carries a variety of vitamin products. Some of these products contain doses far above those necessary in human nutrition, and "megavitamin" therapy is even promoted by physicians. One result has been the promotion of "stress" vitamin products. The following comments by Herbert[91] show the fallacy of this:

> A number of multivitamin "stress" products are advertised for the treatment of alleged vitamin deficiencies and conditions associated with stress, such as surgery, trauma, debilitating infections, and extensive burns. The concept and formulation for these products appears to be adopted largely from a 1952 report on therapeutic nutrition by two nutrition scientists. (Pollack H, Halpren SR: *Therapeutic Nutrition*, publication 234. Washington, DC, Food and Nutrition Board, National Research Council, National Academy of Sciences, 1952). This advertising is deceptive because it does not inform the

13

reader that the Food and Nutrition Board, in an April 1955 release, repudiated allegations that the report contained "recommendations for 'stress formulas'" and pointed out, "The conjectural nature of the report is indicated by the concluding statement in the text" that the recommendations "should be considered tentative pending further research results," and "further research results now indicate the need for critical reconsideration of the subject, and [the Board] has given instructions to withhold further printing and public distribution of publication 234."

In the following discussion, we will consider the toxic effects that have been reported from large doses of vitamins.

Vitamin A　　Overdosage may cause redness and thickening of the skin, blurred vision, and drowziness. Doses in excess of 1 mg (approximately 3,000 International Units) per kg of body weight per day are likely to be toxic. Natural foodstuffs known to contain toxic amounts of this vitamin are the livers of polar bears and fish.

Three studies have shown that massive doses of Vitamin A (as "megavitamin therapy") may cause a serious and easily overlooked disorder in infants and children.[122,127,167] In the five cases reported, the usual symptoms were irritability, vomiting, edema, fever, bone pain and tenderness, and increased intracranial pressure.

Vitamin D　　Overdosage with vitamin D can cause idiopathic hypercalcemia in infancy, even at the recommended dose of 400 International Units per day. The Committee on Nutrition of the American Academy of Pediatrics has set a dose of 1,000 to 3,000 IU/kg body weight/day as dangerous. The symptoms of hypercalcemia are anorexia, vomiting, irritability, constipation, weight loss, and failure to thrive. Mental retardation and death may result.

Because of such devastating reactions to vitamins A and D, the Food and Drug Administration attempted to limit their use. But, says White,[210] "In June of this year [1977], the Second Court of Appeals removed the lid on vitamins A and D so securely placed, we thought, by the Food and Drug Administration. . . . Who now is to protect the consumer from the health food entrepreneur? Segments of that industry successfully challenged the FDA's action, and the constraints against excessive amounts of vitamins A and D are now in jeopardy."

Nicotinic acid and nicotinamide　　Side effects of large doses of these vitamins listed by Herbert[91] include liver damage, severe dermatoses, and peptic ulceration.

Vitamin E　　In two reviews of the adverse effects of large doses of vitamin E, a surprisingly wide variety of side effects has been reported.[90,154] They are summarized in Table 2-1.

Table 2-1
Clinical Disorders Attributed to Vitamin E

Thrombophlebitis

Pulmonary embolism

Hypertension

Fatigue

Gynecomastia and breast tumors

Vaginal bleeding

Headache

Dizziness

Nausea, diarrhea, and intestinal cramps

Muscle weakness and a myopathy (accompanied by elevated serum creatinine kinase levels and creatinuria)

Visual complaints (large doses of vitamin E can antagonize the action of vitamin A)

Hypoglycemia

Stomatitis

Chapping of lips

Urticaria

Apparent aggravation of diabetes mellitus

Apparent aggravation of angina pectoris

Disturbances of reproduction

Decreased rate of wound healing (in experimental animals)

From Roberts HJ: Perspective on vitamin E as therapy. *JAMA* 1981;246:129–130. Courtesy of publisher and author. Copyright 1981, American Medical Association.

Vitamin K   This vitamin is thought to be important in preventing hypoprothrombinemia and hemorrhagic disease of the newborn. Paradoxically, it may cause red-cell hemolysis with overloading of the immature liver with bilirubin and kernicterus. The original fat-soluble type is safest.

Ascorbic acid   The current fad of using huge doses of this vitamin is not without danger. It is thought that the resultant increase in excretion of oxalic acid and uric acid may enhance formation of oxalate or urate crystals to produce kidney and bladder stones.[86]

It has been shown that high doses of ascorbic acid may precipitate gout in susceptible patients.[90] Herbert reports that such doses may cause hemolytic crises in patients with either glucose-6-phosphate dehydrogenase deficiency or sickle cell anemia.[90]

Niacin   High doses of niacin may cause vasodilatation of the skin, headache, abdominal cramps, and nausea. If this usage is prolonged, it may result in an increased frequency of cardiac arrhythmias.

Thiamine   Injections of 10 mg of thiamine have been known to produce anaphylactic shock and vasodilatation.

Hayes and Hegsted have been unable to find evidence of untoward reactions to the other vitamins: pantothenic acid, pyridoxine, choline, and folic acid.[86] But the lesson is clear. Excessive use of vitamin supplements either on an over-the-counter basis or as a "megavitamin" method of treatment may be dangerous.

Seafood Poisoning

In many parts of the world, seafood poisoning is a serious public health problem.[161] At times toxicity is due to microorganisms eaten by the marine animal, the most common being algae and plankton. Seafood likely to be made toxic by the organisms they consume are certain true fish, clams, scallops, and mussels. At other times the fish or other type of seafood is itself toxic. Unfortunately, toxins are not destroyed either by cooking or by the digestive enzymes.

Ciguatera poisoning   In the Caribbean Sea and much of the Pacific Ocean, the disease ciguatera has long been known to exist. It may be caused by the eating of any one of some 350 species of shallow-water fish which, it is thought, become diseased by consuming smaller fish which have fed on toxic algae or plankton. Although mortality rates are not high, death may occur from cardiovascular collapse. Methods of prevention have not proved effective.

Pufferfish poisoning   This problem is confined mainly to Japan and surrounding areas. The toxic factor, produced by the fish itself, is found in certain visceral glands. The Japanese government licenses experts to remove the responsible glands in such a way that the meat of the fish is not contaminated. There are about 100 fatalities per year, most of which are the result of carelessness or ignorance in dressing the fish.

Other marine animal poisons are found in certain herring-like fish of the Pacific, snake mackerels, sharks, dogfish, lampreys, hagfishes, porpoises, and turtles. It is assumed that the poisons are produced by the animals themselves. Of the types of fish poisoning that appear in fish after being cooked, botulism is the most serious.

Trace Elements in Foods

Aluminum   Although high doses of aluminum salts are capable of causing gastrointestinal irritation and rickets (by interfering with phosphate absorption), the amounts present in foods absorbed from aluminum cookware are far too small to be significant.

Arsenic   Poisoning from arsenic may result from accidental, suicidal, or homicidal ingestion of such compounds as calcium arsenate, lead arsenate, or copper arsenate. The three are common insecticides, but since they are poorly absorbed by plants and rapidly excreted by animals, they are no problem in agricultural products. Arsenic is present, however, in some seafood in sufficient concentration to cause poisoning. Its use in therapeutics is now limited.

Iron   According to Underwood, "Iron absorption in normal healthy humans is regulated so efficiently in accordance with body iron needs that intakes from natural foods of sufficient magnitude to produce toxic effects are inconceivable.[200] Over-dosage of ferrous sulfate, however, is a common cause of serious poisoning.

Selenium   According to Bell, the symptoms of selenium poisoning include dermatitis, fatigue, dizziness, and loss of hair and nails.[14] In both the United States and Colombia such cases have been traced to high concentrations of selenium in homegrown foods. Recovery follows a selenium-free diet. A high incidence of gastrointestinal disturbances and icteroid discoloration of the skin is found in areas of the country where the soil is high in selenium. There is also evidence that dental caries are more common in these areas.

Lead   Lead poisoning is a common and serious problem, but retention of lead in plant and animal foods is negligible. However, lead residues from food containers, cups, and dishes may cause poisoning.[50]

Cobalt   Salts of cobalt added to beer to improve its foaming qualities have been incriminated in several epidemics of cardiac failure in heavy beer drinkers. The cobalt and alcohol seem to exert a synergistic effect.[200]

Mercury   In the early 1950s, 50 persons died in Japan from "Minamata disease," caused by high levels of mercury in fish and shellfish taken from Minamata Bay.[200] The outbreak was traced to large amounts of methylmercury in the waste effluents from a plastic factory. In Canada and the United States the maximum permissible level of mercury in fish has been placed at 0.5 parts per million. The maximum acceptable overall dietary concentration has been set at 0.05 parts per million.

Fluorine   Fluoride toxicity may be important in areas where the level in water is extremely high.

Iodide   Although in many parts of the world iodine is useful in the prevention of goiter, it may cause thyrotoxicosis in patients with preexisting goiter. Iodine is found in many foods, but the levels in seafood, iodized salt, and seaweed are especially high.

Underwood finds the following trace elements in foods to be of no real importance as toxicants: copper, molybdenum, zinc, nickel, manganese, tin, cadmium, and chromium.[200]

Lathyrism

In times of famine, peoples of the subcontinent of India and, to some extent, other parts of the world may be obliged to subsist on the seeds of *Lathyrus,* a legume genus that includes the sweet pea. The symptoms include muscular weakness, paralysis of the legs, and, in extreme cases, death. The seeds seem to be harmless when included in a well-balanced diet.

Milk Sickness

This disease is caused by drinking the milk or eating the meat of cattle that have been fed on a common late-summer weed, white snake root, *Eupatorium rugosum.* Although it was once a scourge of the Midwest, milk sickness is now rarely encountered. The symptoms are headache, fatigue, tremor, and collapse. Death was common in the era when the disease was prevalent, and it is said to have caused the death of the mother of Abraham Lincoln. Hartman et al reported a case in 1963.[85]

Pesticides

A variety of chemicals is used to control such agricultural pests as bacteria, fungi, insects, and rodents. By preventing losses in fruits, grains, and vegetables (and indirectly in animal foods), they not only keep down the cost of foods but play an important role in preventing starvation. In recent years considerable anxiety has arisen in the public mind as to the possible toxicity of traces found in foods. Governmental agencies everywhere are concerned with this problem and issue guidelines as to which chemicals may or may not be used. It is now generally agreed that fresh vegetables and fruits are safe as long as they are washed before being eaten. As Coon says, toxins found naturally in foods are much more likely to be harmful than are traces of pesticides.[35]

As to DDT, a pesticide under close scrutiny and whose use is carefully restricted, the *British Medical Journal* has this to say:

> It would be difficult to find a case of dying from D.D.T. and fairly easy to show that this chemical has saved about 10 million lives in

malaria-eradication campaigns alone. Restrictions on D.D.T. (no government has actually banned it) have been largely made to protect wildlife and on general grounds of environmental sanitation. This policy is sensible for the more affluent countries with temperate climates, where insect-borne disease is negligible and few people are starving. But in tropical countries insecticides still offer the only feasible method of reducing numerous insect-borne diseases and protecting crops at a reasonable cost.[55]

Quail poisoning   A rare type of poisoning may be caused by the eating of quails of the Mediterranean area. As Van Veen points out, this is perhaps the earliest reported example of food poisoning.[203] We read in the Book of Numbers, 11:31–33 (New English Bible): "Then a wind from the Lord sprang up; it drove quails from the west, and they were flying all round the camp for the distance of a day's journey, three feet above the ground. . . The people were busy gathering quails all that day, all night, and all the next day. . . But the meat was scarcely between their teeth, and they had not so much as bitten it, when the Lord's anger broke out against the people and he struck them with a deadly plague." It is now recognized that the source of this poisoning is the seeds of poison hemlock *(Conium maculatum)* sometimes eaten by the quails of that part of the world. This is the same hemlock used in the execution of Socrates. Even the biblical report that the birds flew about "three feet above the ground" is supported by modern observation.

Carcinogens

Perhaps no subject is more controversial, confusing, and emotionally charged than the possible carcinogenicity of food products. Animal studies have shown that chemicals, both those naturally present in foods and those added, can, at least in massive dosage, cause both benign and malignant tumors. Miller writes, "Although some of these substances occur in certain common human foods, they have been found primarily in unusual food sources and in foods contaminated by certain fungi. It is virtually certain that other naturally occurring compounds with carcinogenic activity exist among the vast number of nonnutritive minor components of common foods."[133] He and other observers agree that available evidence establishes the safety of foods containing minute amounts of such substances. And the government agencies charged with the responsibility of watching for carcinogenic food additives show extreme caution by forbidding any that are under even the least suspicion. An example of this is the current controversy over saccharin. An order that its use would no longer be allowed in most products was issued by the Food and Drug Administration, to take effect in mid-1977. This was based on Canadian studies indicating that enormous doses appear to cause bladder cancer in rats. Because of strenuous objections to the ban, however, a moratorium was put into effect, which has been extended to mid-1982.

In a thoughtful survey of this problem Roe closes with this comment:

> I believe that it will never be possible to devise a human diet that is entirely free of carcinogenic risk. I therefore suggest that future decisions should be based on assessments of relative safety and relative risk. Common sense as well as data from animal studies should be used to devise a dietary for humans that carries the least overall carcinogenic risk from all sources—food constituents as well as additives and contaminants. The present preoccupation with new chemical additives to the exclusion of natural food constituents and natural contaminants is illogical if not absurd. Testing is expensive and facilities for it are limited. It is important that the limited resources for testing are used in the ways most likely to reduce the overall human cancer burden, but this should not be done without recognizing that malnutrition and famine constitute far worse dangers than cancer in many parts of the world.[155]

Toxic Honey

Most honey in the United States comes from legumes, especially clovers and alfalfa. In some parts of the world bees visit plants containing toxins, and poisoning may be serious.[144] Among plants known to be the source of poisonous honey are mountain laurel, rhododendron, oleander, and azalea.

Miscellaneous toxins   From time to time, poisoning follows ingestion of plant and animal products that are obviously unfit for human consumption. Poisoning by plants is common in young children; the most common offenders found in the United States are listed in Table 2-2. Fortunately, poison-control centers are now to be found in many areas, and information is available by telephone on toxic plants and the treatment indicated for the poisoning they may cause.

Of historical interest is the outbreak of poisoning of the 1930s caused by Jamaica ginger adulterated with tri-ortho-cresyl-phosphate.[135] Sporadic outbreaks still occur from ingestion of lubricating oils containing this poison.[43]

Plant poisoning in adults may be caused by any toxic plant but is most commonly caused by poisonous mushrooms (toadstools). With re-

Table 2-2
Common American Poisonous Plants

Bittersweet (berry)	Narcissus
Blue bonnet	Oleander
Burning bush	Pimpernel
Castor bean	Pink (seed)
Columbine (berry)	Poison hemlock
Cyclamen (tuber)	Pokeweed
Dumb cane	Potato (sprouts)
Elephant ear (bulb)	Rhododendron
Four o'clock	Scotch broom (seed)
Foxglove (leaf)	Spanish bayonet (root)
Iris (rootstock)	Spider lily (bulb)
Jimson weed	Sweet pea (stem)
Lily of the valley	Tulip (bulb)
Mock orange (fruit)	Water hemlock
Monkshood (root)	White snake root
Mountain laurel	

cent interest in "natural foods," persons who experiment with strange plants and strange methods of preparation of ordinary foods may become seriously ill. An example is poisoning involving a group of people who experimented with uncooked beans, well-known sources of phytohemagglutinins.[149]

A curious example of poisoning by ingestion of animal toxins is that caused by eating a newt *(Taricha granulosa)* "on a dare." Of the two cases reported, one terminated in death.[21]

Foods Difficult to Digest

When considering food allergy or any other form of food intolerance, we need to remember that foods vary greatly in digestibility. Among some foods especially difficult to digest for many people, and if they eat enough, *all* people, are: apple, raw melons (including cucumbers), onion, garlic, boiled cabbage, coconut, coffee, pineapple, and most spices. In 1921 the pioneer allergist W. W. Duke recognized the difficulty of distinguishing between gastrointestinal allergy and simple indigestion. He wrote:

> The diagnosis may be doubly difficult because of the fact that the gastrointestinal mucous membrane, when in a chronically reactive

state, is often irritable, with the result that rough or stimulating foods, such as coarse vegetables, fruits, and nuts, condiments, and alcohol, irritate the stomach and augment the symptoms. This usually leads a patient to place the blame for his trouble on foods of this variety rather than on the primary offenders, milk or eggs.[54]

Some foods cause digestive trouble because of fermentation in the lower ileum and colon, especially the colon. The resultant cramping, distension, and flatulence may be severe. Patwardhan has written an interesting review of this problem.[144] He reports that the apparent cause of flatulence associated with mature beans and peas is their high content of trisaccharides and tetrasaccharides. Enzymes are not available for degradation of these more complex carbohydrates. As a result the aerobic and anaerobic bacteria in the ileum and colon bring about fermentation with the production of gases, chiefly methane. Hydrogen, carbon dioxide, ammonia, hydrogen sulfide, indole, skatole, and butyric and valeric acids are also produced. These products account for the foul odor of flatus.

Intolerance to foods that are more or less indigestible is especially common in the elderly and, of course, in those with organic disorders of the gastrointestinal tract such as peptic ulcer, dumping syndrome, esophageal hiatal hernia, and polyposis. At times it is difficult to determine whether the patient's gastrointestinal reaction to a food is caused by allergy, indigestibility, or organic disease. In no type of allergy must differential diagnosis be more carefully done than in gastrointestinal allergy.

Idiosyncrasy

The term *food idiosyncrasy* is now used to refer to non-allergic reactions to wholesome foods. A number of mechanisms may be at work, and some of them, such as those responsible for caffeine intolerance and alcohol intolerance, are not understood.

Favism   Until comparatively recent times, hemolytic anemia resulting from eating the broad, or fava, bean *Vicia faba* was considered an allergic reaction. It is now well established that it is due to deficiency of the enzyme glucose-6-phosphate dehydrogenase.[144] The deficiency is inherited as a sex-linked recessive trait. Vicine, a nucleoside, is thought to be the factor that initiates the reaction. Favism occurs principally in the countries that border the Mediterranean Sea, the highest incidence being in Sardinia. Hemolysis may also be induced in susceptible patients by drugs; the most common are the antimalarials, sulfonamides, nitrofurans, antipyretics, analgesics, sulfones, and vitamin K analogs.

Phenylketonuria The congenital absence of phenylalanine hydroxylase may result in mental deficiency, decreased pigmentation, eczema, and convulsions. Restriction of the diet of such patients to foods low in phenylalanine results in improved growth, development, and mental activity. Several other diseases are caused by deficiency of enzymes whose function is degradation of amino acids. Also of occasional occurrence are congenital deficiency of the digestive enzymes lactase, isomaltase, enterokinase, and sucrase. The possibility of a deficiency of these enzymes should be considered in infants suspected of having digestive disorders of allergic origin.

Drug-induced monoamine oxidase deficiency The function of monoamine oxidase (MAO) is the deamination of naturally occurring amines. It has been found that drugs that inhibit its action are useful in the treatment of depression, the most common drugs being isocarboxazid (Marplan), nialamide (Niamid), phenelzine sulfate (Nardil), and tranylcypromine sulfate (Parnate). Pargyline hydrochloride (Eutonyl) is used to some extent in the treatment of hypertension.

Since patients taking monoamine oxidase inhibitors do not metabolize vasoactive amines, the presence of these agents in foods may cause hypertensive crisis. Among the many vasoactive amines present in foods, tyramine seems to be the one the patient needs to avoid. These are the manufacturer's instructions to patients taking Nardil:

> All patients should be warned against eating foods with high tyramine content (aged cheeses, wines, beer, pickled herring, broad bean pods, chicken liver, yeast extract); any high protein food that is aged or undergoes breakdown by putrefaction process to improve flavor is suspect of being able to produce a hypertensive crisis in patients taking MAO inhibitors; against drinking alcoholic beverages; and against self-medication with certain proprietary agents such as cold, hay fever, or reducing preparations while undergoing Nardil therapy. Beverages containing caffeine may be used in moderation.

The warnings against drugs are directed toward such sympathomimetic (adrenergic) products as phenylephrine (Neo-synephrine), ephedrine, phenylpropanolamine (Propadrine), amphetamines, and isoproterenol.

Celiac disease Celiac disease, the most common type of malabsorption syndrome, was first described in children but also occurs in adults. The exact cause has not been determined, but it is clear that symptoms are brought on by ingestion of gluten. Abnormally large amounts of fat appear in the stools of affected patients, and the absorption of amino acids, dextrose, and fat-soluble vitamins is impaired. Since wheat is the chief source of gluten, celiac disease and true wheat allergy are easily confused.

Monosodium glutamate intolerance Certain susceptible individuals react adversely to the food additive monosodium glutamate, widely used in Chinese and other Oriental cookery. The symptoms are variable, the most common being numbness of the neck, lacrimation, headache. syncope, sweating, dizziness, tachycardia, and paresthesias. Intolerance seems to be related to dose.

Intolerance to monosodium glutamate was first suspected by Man-Kwok, a physician. After eating Chinese food he noticed numbness of the back of the neck and arms, weakness, and palpitation.[128] The syndrome is known as the Chinese restaurant syndrome.[108] (See also Monosodium Glutamate, Chapter 5.)

BACTERIAL FOOD POISONING

Staphylococcal Food Poisoning

An enterotoxin-forming strain of *Staphylococcus aureus* is the most common cause of food poisoning. Since, as Diefenbach has pointed out, this organism can be cultured from about half the population, it is a constant threat. It grows readily in milk and creamed foods, meat, and poultry. Most cases are traced to foods that have been allowed to cool slowly after cooking and to remain for several hours at room temperature. The symptoms include vomiting, abdominal cramps, and diarrhea. Complete recovery usually occurs.

Clostridium Perfringens Poisoning

According to Diefenbach, about one third of reported food poisonings are caused by *Clostridium perfringens*, Type A.[51] The usual source is a meat or poultry dish that has not been cooked at a temperature high enough to kill the spores. Since the toxin is heat-labile, thorough cooking will destroy it. The symptoms are cramps, diarrhea, nausea, and vomiting. The poisoning is usually self-limited.

Botulism

Clostridium botulinum is responsible for the most dreaded type of food poisoning, botulism. Most cases follow the eating of improperly prepared home-canned vegetables. The outstanding symptoms are diplopia, inability to accommodate, dysphagia, dry throat, dysphonia, difficult breathing, and muscular weakness. The immediate threat to life is respiratory failure, and the mortality rate is high. Diefenbach makes these strong recommendations as to prevention:

> Any food removed from a can, particularly home canned, should never be eaten before it has been boiled for at least 20 minutes and thoroughly mixed while cooking. Toxins are susceptible to heat but are not destroyed when foods are merely warmed. A canned food having a disagreeable odor or showing gas pressure should never be tasted. Punctured or bulging cans or jars with defective seals should always be discarded.[51]

Other bacteria which can cause food poisoning are *Bacillus cereus,* group D streptococcus, *Escherichia coli, Proteus,* and *Pseudomonas.* The reactions to the toxins of these organisms are not usually severe.

3 • MANIFESTATIONS OF FOOD ALLERGY

Food allergy may cause a long list of complaints, most of which are subjective and many, bizarre. A patient may have so many complaints, in fact, that he gives the false impression of being neurotic. This is a typical example:

> A woman in her thirties comes in because of nasal congestion, "postnasal drip," fullness of the ears, and frontal headache. When questioned as to other symptoms, she turns out to have many. But, as she says, "All tests were negative and the doctor says it's my nerves." Her other problems include anxiety, fatigue, insomnia, abdominal distress and bloating, alternating diarrhea and constipation, achiness, and recurrent sick headache.

Although in such a case many causative factors, including psychogenic factors, may be at work, both food and inhalant allergy should be considered as the possible source of all her complaints. Food allergy is especially important.

This chapter will outline, system by system, the manifestations of food allergy as they occur in children and adults. The clinical picture in infants, which is in many ways different, is discussed in Chapter 9.

THE RESPIRATORY TRACT

Nasal Allergy

Whether it is called perennial nasal allergy, perennial allergic rhinitis, or vasomotor rhinitis, this is by far the most common allergic disorder. It is seldom caused by foods alone, pollens, molds, epidermals, and house dust being much more important. In cases caused primarily by inhalants, the prominent symptoms are sneezing, nasal itching, nasal discharge, and conjunctivitis. In cases caused primarily by foods, blocking, frontal headache, and increased pharyngeal mucus are the outstanding symptoms. In many cases there is a disagreeable odor to the breath, which the patient may notice himself and complain about bitterly.

Bronchial Allergy

When we think of bronchial allergy, we think chiefly of asthma, the most important of the allergic diseases. In cases caused by food allergy, there is usually not only wheezing and dyspnea but cough with expectoration.[105] In some cases the production of secretions is so great that it is a serious factor in bronchial obstruction.

Some patients with bronchial allergy caused by foods do not wheeze or have noticeable dyspnea. Such patients are often subject to recurrent and prolonged bronchitis. Recurrent pneumonia may also occur but it is much less common. The importance of allergy as a contributing factor in recurrent lower respiratory infection (in both children and adults) is commonly overlooked.

Secretory Otitis Media

One of the most important allergic diseases of children is secretory (or serous) otitis media. It is easily overlooked because the child seldom complains of earache and also because his loss of hearing is usually so slight that it is easily missed by the parents. Whether secretory otitis media is basically an allergic disorder is not known, but allergy is certainly an important factor.[118,125,145,220]

I have found that milk is by far the most common allergen in secretory otitis media in infants and children; it is an occasional cause in adults. The importance of milk as a cause has also been stressed by Phillips,[145] Ziering,[219] Glaser,[73] and Deamer et al.[41]

GASTROINTESTINAL TRACT

Although they commonly occur together, food allergy and gastrointestinal allergy are not the same thing. A patient may have severe food allergy without any gastrointestinal reaction whatever. On the other hand, when gastrointestinal manifestations are caused by allergy, the responsible allergens are almost always an ingested food, drug, or beverage. An exception is an anaphylactic reaction to an injectant that causes vomiting, cramping, and diarrhea.

Abdominal Pain

Next to headache, abdominal pain is probably the most common complaint of both allergic and nonallergic patients. It can be caused by such varied diseases as dysmenorrhea, intercostal neuralgia, peptic ulcer, cholecystitis, gynecologic disease, and countless more. When considering allergy as a possible cause, I always caution the patient that allergy *may* be a cause. He, himself, needs to be alert to other possibilities.

Many times the pain caused by food allergy covers the entire abdomen, varying in degree and in location from one time to the next.[54] It is in this type of case that the patient appears to be (and is often called) neurotic. When pain is localized, it tends to be in the area around the umbilicus, in one of the upper quadrants (more commonly the right), or in the right side and flank.[191]

The patient often has a palpable and tender ascending colon. Some patients say that the sensation is less an aching than a sense of fullness. Two men said it felt as if someone had filled a long balloon with water and placed it upright in the right side.

The patient with aching in the upper abdomen often places his fingertips just under the rib margin. When I see a patient do this, I wonder if the term hypochondriac may not arise from the fact that unexplained pain in the hypochondrium has traditionally been considered a neurosis.

When abdominal pain due to food allergy settles in the right upper quadrant, the clinical picture may be similar to that of gall bladder disease. An occasional patient finds that the pain radiates to the back of the chest, and some cases are accompanied by the passage of clay-colored stools.[191] The clinical evidence is strong that cases of this type represent some sort of involvement of the liver or biliary system. The severe pain of biliary colic with jaundice and dark urine that accompanies obstruction by a common duct stone does not occur.

In 1850 there appeared an interesting article on "dyspepsia," which suggests that the author suspected that milk might cause symptoms referable to the liver or biliary tract:

> Under the influence of milk, used largely by an adult not accustomed to it, the biliary secretion, or at least the excretion of bile, seems to become nearly or wholly suspended, the liver tumefies, and a mild form of jaundice ensues; the eyes, and even the skin, assume a yellow hue; the tongue is coated with a yellow fur; the stools are pale. . . . Popular wisdom explains all this by saying curtly that milk is bilious.[49]

Diarrhea

Diarrhea from food allergy may occur at any time of life but is especially common in children of preschool age. And since these children may not be as well toilet trained as might be desired, diarrhea is a problem not only to the child but to his parents. In older children and adults diarrhea is more of a nuisance than anything else, making it necessary for the patient to be careful about not being too far away from the bathroom at any given time. In severe cases of food allergy the stools may be watery, but they are more likely to be "mushy."

Constipation

To the patient, the word constipation may mean that bowel movements do not occur daily at a regular time. Television commercials and newspaper and magazine advertisements have successfully propagated this misapprehension. But most patients know that the term refers to a condition characterized by hard, lumpy, and often large stools. Constipation is an important symptom of food allergy. That milk is an extremely common cause is well known to patients, although they often believe it is only boiled milk or cheese that causes trouble.

Distension

Abdominal distension, or bloating, is a fairly common manifestation of food allergy.[191] Since the term "bloating" is also applied to fluid retention, and since the term "distension" is not familiar to the uninitiated, it may be necessary to question the patient carefully about his annoying condition. In young children it may be severe enough to cause slight lordosis. Adults may notice that their clothing is often unusually tight. The woman patient comes home and takes off her girdle. The man patient comes home, sits in his easy chair, and loosens his belt and zipper.

Vomiting

Vomiting is not a common manifestation of food allergy in older children or adults, but in infants it is both common and important (see also Food Allergy in Infancy, Chapter 9). Older patients soon learn to avoid any food that causes such an obvious reaction.

Colitis

If asked which manifestation of food allergy is most commonly overlooked, most allergists would probably have difficulty deciding between headache and colitis. Traditionally, any form of colitis not caused by microorganisms, amebic colitis for example, has been considered "functional," in other words, psychosomatic. This is true whether the diagnosis is spastic, mucous, or ulcerative colitis. Many such cases are due to food allergy.

All so-called functional colitis is not of allergic origin, but much of it is. If the patient is prone to abdominal pain, distension, diarrhea, constipation, and the passage of mucus in the stools (or any combination thereof), allergy is a strong possibility. If the symptoms suggest ulcerative colitis, the role of allergy should also be considered. Every case of ulcerative colitis or suspected ulcerative colitis should have an allergic workup, and it should be done early in the course of the disease.[126,150,196]

Pruritus Ani

Among the several possible causes of this annoying, often agonizing dermatitis is food allergy. It should be suspected in any patient who has other symptoms from foods.[191]

Friend, a proctologist, suggests that common causes are coffee, tea, cola drinks, beer, chocolate, and tomato.[69] I am more impressed with the importance of milk, black pepper, and citrus fruits, but no food is above suspicion.

Miscellaneous

Other gastrointestinal disorders that may be caused by foods are aphthous stomatitis (canker sores),[191,198] geographic tongue, and cheilitis. Fetor oris, variously referred to as halitosis, unpleasant breath, or heavy breath, is a common symptom of food allergy.[121,153,191] Sometimes the patient recognizes the offending food, remarking, perhaps, "If I eat an egg, I keep tasting it all day."

THE SKIN
Eczema

In infancy, eczema (atopic dermatitis) has long been recognized as a common and serious manifestation of food allergy. It tends to disappear by the third year but may continue into later childhood and adult life. Whereas in infants the most severe involvement is usually the face, in older patients the common sites are the arm and leg folds, external ear, and neck. Inhalant allergy, incidentally, is a widely overlooked and important cause of eczema in older children and adults.

Urticaria

Knowing that foods are common causes of hives, every new patient and his family have already racked their brains to detect the culprit.

Angioedema

Angioedema (angioneurotic edema) is similar to urticaria but involves deeper vasculature and causes far more swelling. There is usually no itching. Since angioedema may involve the glottis, it is to be taken seriously. Angioedema and urticaria often occur in the same patient.

Purpura

As early as 1914 Osler suggested that vascular purpura of the Henoch-Schonlein type might be due to anaphylaxis, and it is still called anaphylactoid purpura.[142] The cases seen in office practice are likely to involve no more than spots of purpura on the extremities, chiefly the legs and thighs. That vascular purpura is related to urticaria is borne out by the fact that the two may occur together. In fact, large urticarial wheals may have a greyish, purpuric appearance that does not fade on pressure.[82]

Fixed Eruptions

As Derbes has pointed out, fixed eruptions, although most commonly caused by drugs, may be caused by foods.[45] We have seen two cases in which the cause proved to be milk.

SYSTEMIC REACTIONS

Most allergic reactions are relatively benign and are for the most part chronic. They can therefore be approached calmly and leisurely. But when least expected, any patient, allergic or otherwise, may suddenly develop an alarming systemic reaction. This is commonly caused by such drugs as penicillin and aspirin, by contrast media and local anesthetics, by insect stings, and even by massive inhalation of potent allergens. It also can be caused by foods, especially such notoriously potent allergens as walnut, buckwheat, cottonseed, fish, peanut, egg, and shrimp.

Acute Asthma

The most common systemic allergic reaction is asthma. Most patients with asthma are careful to avoid the offending allergens, including foods, but sometimes a potent allergen is eaten accidentally.

Every allergist knows of children who have been compelled to eat a food to which they are extremely allergic. I well remember a teacher telling one of my asthmatic children that a little of the chocolate cake wouldn't hurt her. I had to see her on an emergency basis.

Edema of the Glottis

As has been mentioned, angioedema involving the glottis may be a serious emergency. It is to be suspected when any patient suddenly complains of swelling of the tongue, hoarseness, or stridor. A school teacher was brought directly from the school in great haste with this emergency. "I forgot," she said, "to ask if there was peanut butter in the homemade cookies another teacher brought."

Anaphylactic Shock

The most serious of all allergic reactions, anaphylactic shock, may be caused by foods. It is especially serious in infants and at that stage of life may be fatal.[47,107,137,209] I have been unable to find instances of foods causing fatal anaphylactic shock in older children and adults.

In 1869 Fergus reported a patient's reaction to strawberry:

"Some strawberry jam was tasted merely on the tip of the finger; in a short time the patient was on the floor, perfectly flaccid, but powerless to move, fainting on the slightest attempt at motion."[46] The patient had always reacted in the same way to strawberry, the attack usually lasting half an hour. Undoubtedly many of these cases are passed off as hysteria, which, of course, they may sometimes be. But any allergist would respect the caution of Fergus, offered over a century ago: "There can be no doubt that in this case a single strawberry might cause death."[61]

Similar cases have been reported from pea and egg. Unquestionably, many go unreported.

GENITOURINARY TRACT

Among the genitourinary disturbances that have been reported from allergy are vulvovaginal irritation, enuresis, frequency and burning on urination, and albuminuria. Patients rarely think of the possibility of an allergic origin of these symptoms and will not mention them unless specifically questioned. These manifestations are seldom caused by food allergy, but if allergy is at fault, nothing else will bring relief.

Albuminuria

In 1941 Danis reported three cases of what appeared to be nephrosis in which allergy to foods seemed to be the cause. Because of the limited number of cases and the fact that a definite cause-and-effect relationship was not established, the study is not convincing.[37]

In 1966 Matsumura et al. studied sixteen cases of typical orthostatic albuminuria. They suspected the role of allergy because the children had such evidence of constitutional allergy as abdominal pain, nausea, headache, and fatigue. By provocative feeding they implicated the following offenders; milk, 9 cases; egg, 2 cases; milk and egg, 2 cases; soybean, 2 cases; and milk, egg, and soybean, 1 case.[130]

Bladder and Urethral Disorders

In 1954 Powell and Powell studied 82 women with lower urinary tract symptoms, including dysuria, frequency, urgency, and recurrent pyuria. Most patients had a history of food allergy.[148] They were able to show that the following foods caused symptoms: citrus fruits, 49 cases; tomato, 28 cases; condiments, 16 cases; chocolate, 13 cases; grape, 12 cases; apple, 7 cases; watermelon, 6 cases.

My own experience is similar to that of Powell and Powell, except that I find milk to be especially common; they reported only 2 cases. As to what they call condiments, I find black pepper to be the most common offender. It is also first on their list.

MUSCULOSKELETAL SYSTEM

Almost all patients with extensive food allergy complain of muscular aching.[175] The most commonly involved muscle groups are those of the neck, upper back, and extremities. It may be severe. Achiness is at times limited to the joints, especially those of the hand, elbow, and knee. Food allergy is a common and almost universally overlooked cause of "growing pains" of childhood.

NERVOUS SYSTEM

Headache

Allergic headache ranges from mild frontal aching to severe classic migraine. The milder type is often referred to as "common migraine." The symptoms other than headache amount to little more than vague nausea and dizziness.

Classic migraine tends to occur sporadically, perhaps every two to three weeks. The pain is characteristically severe, throbbing, and often prostrating. Systemic symptoms include nausea, vomiting, scintillating scotoma, feelings of unreality, paresthesias, anesthesias, and vertigo.

Whatever the patient's presenting complaint, every type of headache should be considered of possible allergic origin.[178-181] This includes common and classic migraine and cluster headache. It should be kept in mind that headache is a common manifestation of food allergy in children. It may begin as early as one year.

The Tension-Fatigue Syndrome

In 1916 Hoobler, a pediatrician, reported that unusual restlessness and sensitivity were common in allergic children and were often the complaints that brought the child to the physician.[94] In 1922, in a more extended study, Shannon confirmed these findings and added several cases of his own.[166] In 1930 Rowe found the same complaints to be common in allergic adults.[157] In 1954, hoping to draw more attention to this problem and to give it its proper status as an allergic disorder, I introduced the term allergic tension-fatigue syndrome.[175]

In the following selections the reader can gain insight into what various observers have thought of these strange allergic symptoms:

Shannon (1922): Eight cases showing marked evidences of the so-called neuropathic diathesis in infants and children have been presented. . . . All showed definite relief from the nervous symptoms on the institution of specific therapy directed at the problem to which they were sensitive.[166]

Wooton (1934): A neurotic young matron, age 31, would have peculiar sensations or feelings after eating. She would become so irritable that at times she would almost lose self-control. . . . Breakfast was all right, but lunch and dinner almost invariably brought on tantrums. . . . Believe it or not, her disposition underwent a complete though slow metamorphosis as the allergic foods were removed from her diet.[217]

Turnbull (1943): Many of these patients, formerly with wonderful dispositions, calm, happy, cheerful, and thoughtful of others, and now in this cloudy, blank, confused condition, become very irritable and miserable and misunderstand the good intentions of family and friends.[199]

Jones (1949): Abnormalities of behavior such as listlessness, easy fatiguability, restlessness, over-activity, stammering, various kinds of nervousness, and inattention often result from food allergy and can be relieved only when the offending foods are eliminated completely.[101]

Davison (1952): The following symptoms have been reported by the writer and others as having been proven to be caused by allergic sensitivity: Emotional and personality changes—increase in temper; screaming attacks; patient is mean or sulky, irritable, whining, impatient, quarrelsome, sensitive, easily hurt, unhappy, morbid, depressed, restless, tense, nervous, jumpy, fearful, anxious, irresponsible, erratic, uncooperative, unpredictable, pugnacious, or cruel; can't be pleased; is not open to reason; cries without cause; worries, feels terrible, contemplates suicide; is nervous and high-strung; chews clothes and bedclothes; has nightmares; loses pride in work, in clothing, and in cleanliness; doesn't care; can't make decisions; loses interest in the opposite sex; has childish compulsions.[40]

Crook (1963): Tension and fatigue are part of a primary allergic disorder of the nervous system. Such a disorder may occur alone, or it may be accompanied by other allergic syndromes such as asthma, hay fever, or eczema. In addition, these and other nervous system symptoms are not necessarily due to the same allergens that cause other allergic conditions.[36]

Leonard, a psychologist (1966): It is important for those who work with children to be aware of the types of behavior manifested by allergic children, such as the types reported. There are probably many times when children and parents are frustrated by unsuccessful psychological and medical treatment when symptoms are not recognized as having an allergic etiology but thought to be the result of some organic or emotional factors.[119]

Wolf (1971): The tension-fatigue syndrome is part of a primary allergic disorder of the nervous system. It may occur alone or in combination with other allergic manifestations. Of interest is the fact that the cause of the patient's typical allergic manifestations may differ from the cause of the tension-fatigue syndrome.[215]

Weinberg and Tuchinda (1973): The allergic tension-fatigue syndrome. . . is seen most frequently in children of all ages but may also occur in adults. . . . Fatigue, or the feeling that the child is "run down" is often the main complaint which prompts the parents to seek medical assistance.[207]

An interesting finding is that the tension-fatigue syndrome is often discovered independently by those who have never heard of it. For example, Murray, a pediatrician, wrote a letter asking if other pediatricians had noticed behavior problems associated with ingestion of milk and dairy products. He reported that the behavior of children is often "totally changed by withholding of dairy products."[138]

Another even more dramatic example was the discovery by a woman that her severely disturbed husband's behavior was caused by milk. Fortunately, the allergist whom she consulted agreed that her observations were correct.[24]

My purpose in giving such extended coverage to the tension-fatigue syndrome is to draw attention to the fact that many children with so-called hyperactivity and many adults with presumed neuroses are actually victims of the subtle allergic condition.

Convulsions

Food allergy can, on rare occasions, result in typical grand mal seizures, a fact little known. Davison was able to collect a total of 57 cases.[40] Whenever a patient has both seizures and evidence of allergy, allergic study is definitely indicated. Because a seizure is so serious a reaction, parents and the physician are unwilling to challenge the patient to establish a definite relationship to food allergy. For this reason, such a relationship must often be surmised rather than proved.

MISCELLANEOUS ALLERGIC MANIFESTATIONS

One of the neglected areas of pediatrics is the role of milk allergy in causing so-called iron-deficiency anemia. In 17 of 34 cases, Wilson et al were able to demonstrate the cause to be blood loss in the stools secondary to milk-induced gastrointestinal allergy. Gryboski, in a study of 21 infants with gastrointestinal allergy, found that all had hypochromic anemia. The average hemoglobin was 9.5 g. The patient with the highest reading was 16 g, but he was badly dehydrated, and when hydrated, his reading dropped promptly to 10 g.

Other minor symptoms of food allergy are fluid retention (especially in women), pallor,[153,175] infraorbital edema and discoloration (first described in 1912 by Schorer,[162] a pediatrician), recurrent croup, excessive sweating and salivation, and chilliness.

One of the unusual manifestations of food allergy is fever.[44,158] It is more common in small children, but as one of my recent cases illustrates, it may persist into later childhood:

> This patient, a 53-year-old woman, is currently under treatment for multiple allergies. She has always disliked eggs, and when made to eat them in childhood would develop chills and fever. At the age of 14, while living in Texas, her cooking class prepared scrambled eggs. When the teacher put forth the rule "we eat what we cook," the patient told her she could not eat eggs. She, however, was made to do so. In about a half hour she began to chill and was allowed to go home. She still remembers sitting in the hot Texas sun trying to stop chilling. Fever ensued in a short time and persisted for two or three days. She remarked, "We lived across the street from the school, and

my mother made sure that the cooking teacher would never again force a child to eat a food that she said she couldn't eat."

At the age of 30 she decided to teach her daughter to cook, and the two made a meat loaf containing two eggs. She ate a small portion. This time she developed cramps, distension, and diarrhea but not fever. She had had similar reactions to hollandaise sauce, mayonnaise, waffles, and pancakes. When given a "flu shot" she developed chills, fever, and prostration. She was confined to her bed for two weeks largely because of persistent and severe muscle cramping.

4 • BIOLOGICAL CLASSIFICATION OF FOODS

Foods are ordinarily classed under such headings as vegetables, fruits, meats, cereals, dairy products, spices, and nuts. We may call this the *conventional classification,* the one used by those who prepare foods and those who eat them. In allergy practice we must use a different classification, one based on botanical and zoological relationships. This is the *biological classification.* Its value depends on the important fact that a food acting as an allergen tends to cross-react with closely related species, i.e., a patient allergic to a given food is likely to be allergic to its close relatives.

The biological classification is especially important in dealing with foods of the vegetable kingdom. Most people include in their diet some 80 to 120 varieties of plants, and there is usually little correspondence between the conventional and biological classifications. Here are examples: buckwheat is related to rhubarb, not wheat; peanut is related to soybean, not pecan; cinnamon is related to avocado, not ginger; almond is related to peach, not walnut; date is related to coconut, not fig; cabbage is related to mustard, not lettuce; spinach is related to beet, not New Zealand spinach; cashew nut is related to mango, not Brazil nut; red pepper is related to potato, not black pepper; potato is related to eggplant, not sweet potato; and strawberry, blueberry, and gooseberry belong to different families.

To illustrate the importance of dropping the conventional classification of foods in allergy practice, let us imagine a botanist ordering a meal in a restaurant. After studying the menu he orders a vegetable plate. When his food arrives, the plate contains stewed tomato, green beans, corn on the cob, squash, eggplant, and okra. The salad is made up of sliced cucumbers and tomato with a dressing made of wine vinegar, olive oil, red pepper, and black pepper. The botanist sits back in his chair, looks up to the waiter and says, "This is not a vegetable plate. These are all fruits."

Both the botanist and the waiter are right. Although the foods involved are botanically classed as fruits, according to modern usage, any plant food served in the main course of a meal is a vegetable. But the allergist must think like the botanist. He is not so much interested in how foods are used as he is in what they are—and in how they are related.

The remainder of this chapter is devoted to three tables. The first two, Tables 4-1 and 4-2, are concerned with plant foods. Table 4-1 is an alphabetical list of the different *plant foods* with the plant food family to which each belongs. Table 4-2 is an alphabetical list of *plant food families* and their members. These tables allow the reader to identify the family to which any plant food belongs. Suppose, for example, that a patient is known to be allergic to thyme. Table 4-1 shows it to be a member of the mint family. The reader can then turn to Table 4-2 and identify the other members of the family.

Table 4-3, the third of the food lists, outlines the relationships of *animal foods*. Since animal foods are relatively few in number and since their relationships are usually obvious, a simple list of the relevant groups is adequate. These groups are listed phylogenetically, ranging from simple invertebrates to mammals. From a practical point of view animal allergens differ from plant allergens in two ways: 1) cross-reactivity is less pronounced, especially in the case of birds and mammals, and 2) when cross-reactivity does exist it usually extends beyond the limits of the biological family to the biological class.

Table 4-1
Plant Foods

Food	Family
Acacia	Mimosa
Ackee	Soapberry
Acorn	Oak
Agar	Seaweed
Alfalfa	Pea
Allspice	Myrtle
Almond	Plum
Ambarella	Cashew
Angelica	Parsley
Anise	Parsley
Annatto	Indian plum
Apple	Apple
Apricot	Plum
Arrowroot	Arrowroot
Artichoke	Sunflower
Asparagus	Lily
Avocado	Laurel
Balm	Mint
Balsam of Peru	Pea
Bamboo	Grass

Table 4-1 *(continued)*

Food	Family
Banana	Banana
Barbados strawberry	Cactus
Barberry	Barberry
Barley	Grass
Basil	Mint
Bay leaf	Laurel
Bean	Pea
Beechnut	Beech
Beet	Goosefoot
Bengal quince	Citrus
Bergamot	Mint
Bilberry	Heath
Bilimbi	Wood sorrel
Black guava	Madder
Blackhaw	Honeysuckle
Black pepper	Pepper
Black sapote	Ebony
Blackberry	Rose
Bladder weed	Seaweed
Blueberry	Heath
Borage	Borage
Boysenberry	Rose
Brazil nut	Brazil nut
Breadfruit	Mulberry
Breadnut	Mulberry
Broccoli	Mustard
Brussels sprouts	Mustard
Buckwheat	Buckwheat
Buffalo berry	Oleaster
Burdock	Sunflower
Burnet	Rose
Butternut	Walnut
Cabbage	Mustard
Cactus	Cactus
Calendula	Sunflower
Camomile	Sunflower
Cantaloupe	Gourd
Cape gooseberry	Nightshade
Caper	Caper
Caraway seed	Parsley
Cardamom	Ginger
Cardoon	Sunflower

Table 4-1 *(continued)*

Food	Family
Carob bean	Pea
Carrageen	Seaweed
Carrot	Parsley
Cashew	Cashew
Cassava	Spurge
Cassia	Laurel
Cauliflower	Mustard
Cayenne pepper	Nightshade
Celeriac	Parsley
Celery	Parsley
Celtuce	Sunflower
Ceriman	Arum
Chayote	Gourd
Cherimoya	Custard apple
Cherry	Plum
Chervil	Parsley
Chestnut	Beech
Chickpea	Pea
Chicle	Sapodilla
Chicory	Sunflower
Chilean guava	Myrtle
Chili pepper	Nightshade
Chinese gooseberry	Actidinia
Chinquapin	Beech
Chives	Lily
Chocolate	Cola
Cinnamon	Laurel
Citron	Citrus
Citron melon	Gourd
Clary	Mint
Cloudberry	Rose
Clove	Myrtle
Clover	Pea
Coca leaf	Coca
Coconut	Palm
Coffee	Madder
Cohune nut	Palm
Cola	Cola
Collards	Mustard
Comino	Parsley
Coriander	Parsley
Corn	Grass

Table 4-1 *(continued)*

Food	Family
Corn salad	Valerian
Costmary	Sunflower
Cottonseed	Mallow
Cowpea	Pea
Cranberry	Heath
Cucumber	Gourd
Cumin	Parsley
Currant	Gooseberry
Custard apple	Custard apple
Dandelion	Sunflower
Dasheen	Arum
Date	Palm
Day lily	Lily
Dill	Parsley
Dock	Buckwheat
Dulse	Seaweed
Durian	Mallow
East Indian arrowroot	Ginger
Eggplant	Nightshade
Elderberry	Honeysuckle
Endive	Sunflower
Feijoa	Myrtle
Fennel	Parsley
Fenuqreek	Pea
Fiddlehead fern	Fern
Fig	Mulberry
Filbert	Birch
Flaxseed	Flax
Florida arrowroot	Cycad
Garbanzo	Pea
Garden cress	Mustard
Garlic	Lily
Ginger	Ginger
Ginkgo	Ginkgo
Gooseberry	Gooseberry
Gooseberry tree	Wood sorrel
Granadilla	Passionflower
Grape	Grape
Grapefruit	Citrus
Ground cherry	Nightshade
Guar	Pea
Guarana	Soapberry

Table 4-1 *(continued)*

Food	Family
Guava	Myrtle
Guava, Chilean	Myrtle
Hackberry	Elm
Hazelnut	Birch
Hickory nut	Walnut
Hop	Mulberry
Horehound	Mint
Horseradish	Mustard
Huckleberry	Heath
Hyssop	Mint
Iceland moss	Lichen
Indian plum	Indian plum
Irish moss	Seaweed
Jackfruit	Mulberry
Jambolan	Myrtle
Japanese artichoke	Mint
Jasmine	Olive
Jerusalem artichoke	Sunflower
Jujube	Buckthorn
Juneberry	Apple
Juniper	Pine
Kaki	Ebony
Kale	Mustard
Karaya gum	Cola
Kiwi fruit	Actidinia
Kohlrabi	Mustard
Kumquat	Citrus
Lamb's quarters	Goosefoot
Lansa	Bead tree
Lavender	Mint
Laver	Seaweed
Leek	Lily
Lemon	Citrus
Lemon verbena	Vervain
Lentil	Pea
Lettuce	Sunflower
Licorice	Pea
Lime	Citrus
Lingonberry	Heath
Litchi	Soapberry
Longan	Soapberry
Loquat	Apple

Table 4-1 *(continued)*

Food	Family
Lotus	Water lily
Lovage	Parsley
Macadamia nut	Protea
Mace	Nutmeg
Maize	Grass
Malay apple	Cashew
Malay plum	Indian plum
Mamey	Mamey
Mango	Cashew
Mango pepper	Nightshade
Mangosteen	Gamboge
Manna	Olive
Manzanilla	Apple
Maple	Maple
Marjoram	Mint
Maté	Holly
Medlar	Apple
Melluco	Goosefoot
Mesquite	Pea
Millet	Grass
Mint	Mint
Mombin	Cashew
Morel	Sac fungi
Mulberry	Mulberry
Mushroom	Mushroom
Mustard	Mustard
Nasturtium	Nasturtium
New Zealand spinach	Carpet weed
Nutmeg	Nutmeg
Oats	Grass
Okra	Mallow
Olive	Olive
Onion	Lily
Orach	Goosefoot
Orange	Citrus
Oregano	Mint
Orris root	Iris
Otaheite apple	Cashew
Oyster plant	Sunflower
Papaw (British)	Papaya
Papaw (US)	Custard apple
Papaya	Papaya

46

Table 4-1 *(continued)*

Food	Family
Paprika	Nightshade
Paradise nut	Brazil nut
Parsley	Parsley
Parsnip	Parsley
Passion fruit	Passionflower
Pea	Pea
Peach	Plum
Peanut	Pea
Pear	Apple
Pecan	Walnut
Pepper, bell (mango)	Nightshade
Pepper, black and white	Pepper
Pepper, red	Nightshade
Peppermint	Mint
Persimmon	Ebony
Pineapple	Pineapple
Pinyon nut	Pine
Pipsissewa	Heath
Pistachio nut	Cashew
Pitaya	Cactus
Plantain	Banana
Plum	Plum
Pokeweed	Pokeweed
Pomegranate	Pomegranate
Popcorn	Grass
Poppyseed	Poppy
Potato	Nightshade
Potato, sweet	Morning glory
Prickly pear	Cactus
Prune	Plum
Pulasan	Soapberry
Pumpkin	Gourd
Purslane	Purslane
Queensland arrowroot	Canna
Quince	Apple
Radish	Mustard
Raisin	Grape
Rambutan	Soapberry
Rapeseed	Mustard
Raspberry	Rose
Rhubarb	Buckwheat
Rice	Grass

Table 4-1 *(continued)*

Food	Family
Rooibusch	Sunflower
Roseapple	Myrtle
Rutabaga	Mustard
Rye	Grass
Safflower	Sunflower
Saffron	Iris
Sage	Mint
Sago	Cycad
Sago palm	Palm
Salep	Orchid
Salsify	Sunflower
Samphire	Parsley
Sapodilla	Sapodilla
Sapote	Sapodilla
Sarsaparilla	Lily
Sassafras	Laurel
Savory	Mint
Sea grape	Buckwheat
Sesame	Sesame
Shallot	Lily
Skirret	Parsley
Sloe	Plum
Sorghum	Grass
Soursop	Custard apple
Soybean	Pea
Spearmint	Mint
Spinach	Goosefoot
Squash	Gourd
Star anise	Parsley
Star apple	Star apple
Strawberry	Rose
Sugar apple	Custard apple
Sugarcane	Grass
Sunflower seed	Sunflower
Surinam cherry	Myrtle
Sweet cicily	Parsnip
Sweet granadilla	Passionflower
Sweet potato	Morning glory
Swiss chard	Goosefoot
Tamarind	Pea
Tangelo	Citrus
Tansy	Sunflower

Table 4-1 *(continued)*

Food	Family
Tapioca	Spurge
Taro	Arum
Tarragon	Sunflower
Tea	Tea
Thyme	Mint
Tomato	Nightshade
Tragacanth	Pea
Truffle	Truffle
Turmeric	Ginger
Turnip	Mustard
Vanilla	Orchid
Vegetable marrow	Gourd
Vine spinach	Basselad
Walnut	Walnut
Water chestnut	Water chestnut
Watercress	Mustard
Watermelon	Gourd
West Indies cherry	Malpighiad
Wheat	Grass
Wild rice	Grass
Wintercress	Mustard
Wintergreen	Heath
Yam	Yam
Yeast	Yeast
Zedoary	Ginger

Table 4-2
Classification of Plant Foods

Family	Plant
Actidinia, *Actidiniaceae*	Docks and sorrels, *Rumex* spp.
	Kiwi fruit, *Actidinia chinensis*
Apple, *Pomaceae*	Apple, *Pyrus malus*
	Crab apple, *Pyrus* spp.
	Juneberry, *Amelanchier canadensis*
	Loquat, *Eriobotrya japonica*
	Manzanilla, *Crataequs* spp.
	Medlar, *Mespilus germanica*
	Pear, *Pyrus communus*
	Quince, *Cydonia oblonga*

Table 4-2 *(continued)*

Family	Plant
Arrowroot, *Marantaceae*	Arrowroot, *Maranta* spp.
Arum, *Araceae*	Ceriman, *Monstera deliciosa*
	Dasheen, *Colocasia* spp.
	Taro, *Colocasia* spp.
Banana, *Musaceae*	Banana, *Musa sapientum*
	Plantain, *Musa paradisiaca*
Barberry, *Berberidaceae*	Barberry, *Berberis vulgaris*
Basselad, *Basseladaceae*	Vine spinach, *Basella alba*
Bead tree, *Maliaceae*	Lansa, *Lansium domesticum*
Beech, *Fagaceae*	Beechnut, *Fagus* spp.
	Chestnut, *Castanea dentata*
	Chinquapin, *Castanea pumila*
Birch, *Betulaceae*	Filbert, *Corylus avellana*
	Hazelnut, *Corylus americana*
Borage, *Boraginaceae*	Borage, *Borago officinalis*
Brazil nut, *Lecythidaceae*	Brazil nut, *Bertholletia excelsa*
	Paradise nut, *Lecythus* spp.
Buckthorn, *Rhamnaceae*	Jujube, *Zizyphys* spp.
Buckwheat, *Polygonaceae*	Buckwheat, *Fagopyrum esculentum*
	Dock, *Rumex* spp.
	Rhubarb, *Rheum rhaponticum*
	Sea grape, *Coccoloba ovifera*

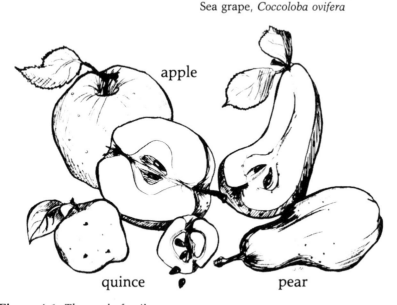

Figure 4-1 The apple family

50

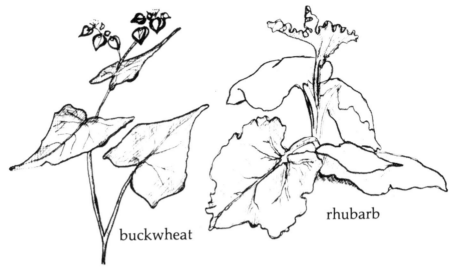

Figure 4-2 The buckwheat family

Table 4-2 *(continued)*

Family	Plant
Cactus, *Cactaceae*	Barbados strawberry, *Pereskia aculeata*
	Pitaya, *Cereus compressus*
	Prickly pear, *Opuntia vulgaris*
Canna, *Cannaceae*	Queensland arrowroot, *Canna edulis*
Caper, *Capparidaceae*	Caper, *Capparis solada*
Carpetweed, *Aizoaceae*	New Zealand spinach, *Tetragonia expansa*
Cashew, *Anacardiaceae*	Ambarella (Otaheite apple), *Spondias Cytheria*
	Cashew, *Anacardium occidentale*
	Mango, *Mangifera indica*
	Pistachio, *Pistacia vera*
	Red mombin, *Spondius mombin*
	Yellow mombin, *Spondius lutea*
Citrus, *Rutaceae*	Bengal quince, *Aegle marmelos*
	Citron, *Citrus medica* var.
	Grapefruit, *Citrus paradisi*
	Kumquat, *Fortunella japonica*
	Lemon lime, *Citrus medica*

Table 4-2 *(continued)*

Family	Plant
	Orange, tangerine, *Citrus aurentium*
	Tangelo, *Citrus paradisis et reticulata*
Coca, Erythrozylaceae	Coca leaf, *Erythlen coca*
Cola nut, *Sterculiaceae*	Chocolate, *Theobroma cacao*
	Cola (kola) nut, *Cola accuminata*
	Karaya gum, *Sterculia urens*
Custard apple, *Annonaceae*	Cherimoya, *Annona cherlmolia*
	Custard apple, *Annona reticulata*
	Pawpaw, *Asimina triloba*
	Soursop, *Annona muricata*
	Sugar apple (sour sop), *Annona sguamosa*
Cycad, *Cycadaceae*	Florida arrowroot, *Zamia florida*
	Sago, *Cycas* spp.
Ebony, *Ebonaceae*	Black sapote, *Diospyros ebenaster*
	Kaki (Japanese persimmon) *Diospyros kaki*

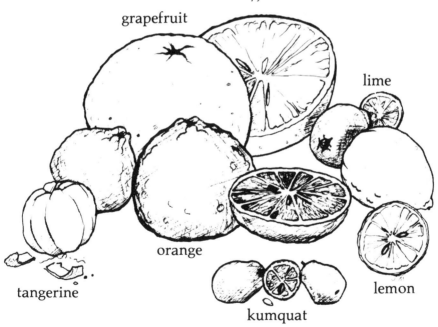

Figure 4-3 The citrus family

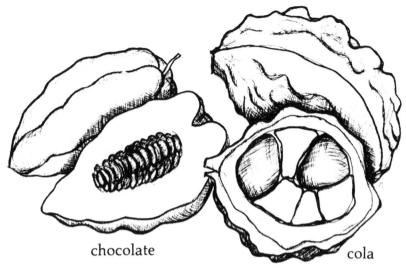

chocolate   cola

Figure 4-4 The cola family

Table 4-2 *(continued)*

Family	Plant
	Persimmon, *Diospyros virginiana*
Elm, *Ulmaceae*	Hackberry, *Celtis occidentalis*
Fern, *Filicales* (order)	Fiddlehead fern, *Osmunda cinnamomea*
Flax, *Linaceae*	Flaxseed, *Linum usitatissimum*
Fungi (various families)	(See Lichen, Mushroom, Sac fungi, Truffle, Yeast families)
Gamboge, *Guttiferae*	Mangosteen, *Garcinia mangostana*
Ginger, *Zingiberaceae*	Cardamom, *Elettaria cardamomum*
	East Indian arrowroot, *Curcuma angustifolia*
	Ginger, *Zingiber officinale*
	Turmeric, *Curcuma longa*
	Zedoary, *Curcuma zedoria*
Ginkgo, *Ginkgoaceae*	Ginkgo, *Ginkgo biloba*
Gooseberry, *Grossulariaceae*	Currant, *Ribes* spp.
	Gooseberry, *Ribes grossularia*
Goosefoot, *Chenopodiaceae*	Beet, *Beta vulgaris*
	Lamb's quarters, *Chenopodium alba*

Table 4-2 *(continued)*

Family	Plant
	Melluco (alluco), *Ullucus tuberosus*
	Orach, *Atriplex hortensis*
	Spinach, *Spinacia oleracea*
	Swiss chard, *Beta cicla*
Gourd, *Cucurbitaceae*	Cantaloupe, *Cucumis melo*
	Chayote, *Sechium edule*
	Chinese watermelon, *Benencasa hispida*
	Citron melon, *Citrullus vulgaris*
	Cucumber, *Cucumis sativus*
	Gherkin, *Cucumis anguria*
	Pumpkin, *Cucurbita pepo*
	Summer squash, *Cucurbita pepo* var.
	Vegetable marrow, *Cucurbita ovifera*
	Watermelon, *Citrullus vulgaris*
	Winter squash, *Cucurbita maxima* and *C. moschata*

Figure 4-5 The goosefoot family

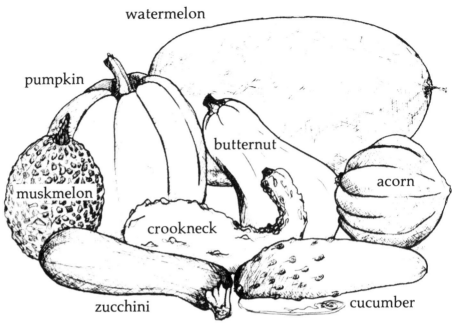

Figure 4-6 The gourd family

Table 4-2 *(continued)*

Family	Plant
Grape, Vitaceae	American grape, *Vitis,* spp.
	European grape, *Vitis vinefera*
Grass, *Gramineae*	Bamboo, *Bambusa* spp.
	Barley, *Hordeum vulgare*
	Corn (maize), *Zea mays*
	Millet, *Panicum, Setaria,* and *Pennisetum* spp.
	Oats, *Avena sativa*
	Popcorn, *Zea mays,* var. *everta*
	Rice, *Oryza sativa*
	Rye, *Secale cereale*
	Sorghum, milo, *Andropogon sorghum*
	Sugarcane, *Saccharum officinarum*
	Wheat, *Triticum sativum*
	Wild rice, *Zizania aguatica*
Heath, *Ericaceae*	Bilberry, *Vaccinium* spp.
	Blueberry, *Vaccinium* spp.
	Cranberry, *Oxycoccus macrocarpon*

Table 4-2 *(continued)*

Family	Plant
	Huckleberry, *Gaylussacia baccata*
	Lingonberry, *Vaccinium vitis-idaea*
	Pipsissewa, *Chimaphila umbellata*
Holly, *Ilicaceae*	Maté (yerba mate), *Ilex paraguariensis*
Honeysuckle, *Caprifoliaceae*	Blackhaw, *Viburnum prunefolium*
	Elderberry, *Sumbucus canadensis*
	Genipap, *Genipa americana*
Indian plum, *Bixaceae*	Annatto (Arnato), *Bixa orellana*
	Indian plum, *Flacourtia cataphracta*
	Malay plum, *Flacourtia ramontchi*
Iris, *Iridaceae*	Orris root, *Iris florentina*
	Saffron, *Crocus sativus*
Laurel, *Lauraceae*	Avocado, *Persea* spp.
	Bay leaf, *Laurus nobilis*

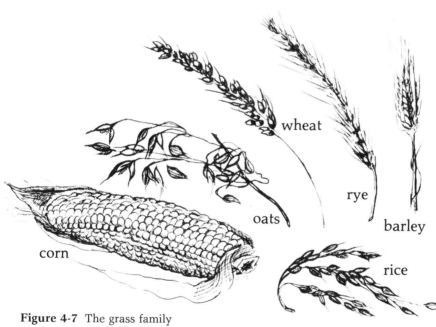

Figure 4-7 The grass family

Table 4-2 *(continued)*

Family	Plant
	Cassia, *Cassia* spp.
	Cinnamon, *Cinnamonum zeylanicum*
	Sassafras, *Sassafras officinale*
Lichen (one family, *Cetrariaceae*)	Iceland moss, *Cetraria islandica*
Lily, *Liliaceae*	Asparagus, *Asparagus officinalis*
	Chives, *Allium schaenoprasum*
	Day lily, *Hemerocallus flava*
	Garlic, *Allium sativum*
	Leek, *Allium porrum*
	Onion, *Allium cepa*
	Sarsaparilla, *Smilax officinalis*
	Shallot, *Allium ascalonicum*
	Welch onion, *Allium fistulosum*
Madder, *Rubiaceae*	Black guava, *Guettanda argentea*
	Coffee, *Caffea* spp.

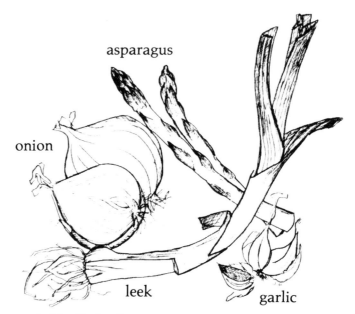

Figure 4-8 The lily family

Table 4-2 *(continued)*

Family	Plant
Magnolia, *Magnoliaceae*	Star anise, *Illicium verum*
Mallow, *Malvaceae*	Cottonseed, *Gossypium* spp.
	Durian, *Durio zibethinus*
	Okra, *Hibiscus esculentus*
Malpighiad, *Malpighidaceae*	West Indian cherry, *Malpighia glabra*
Mamey, *Clusiaceae*	Mamey, *Mammea americana*
Maple, *Aceraceae*	Maple, *Acer* spp.
Mimosa, *Mimosaceae*	Acacia, *Acacia senegal*
Mint, *Labiatae*	Balm, *Melissa officinalis*
	Basil, *Osimum basilicum*
	Bergamot, *Mentha canadensis*
	Clary, *Salvia sclarea*
	Horehound, *Marrubium vulgare*
	Hyssop, *Hyssopus officinalis*
	Japanese artichoke, *Stachus seiboldi*
	Lavender, *Lavendula vera*
	Marjoram, *Origanum* spp
	Oregano, *Lippia palmeri*
	Peppermint, *Mentha piperita*
	Sage, *Salvia officinalis*
	Savory, *Satureia hortensis*
	Spearmint, *Mentha spicata*
	Thyme, *Thymus vulgaris*
Morning glory, *Convolvulaceae*	Sweet potato, *Ipomoca batatas*
Mulberry, *Moraceae*	Breadfruit, *Brosium alicastrum*
	Fig, *Ficus carica*
	Hop, *Humulus iupulus*
	Jackfruit, *Artocarpus integrifolia*
	Mulberry, *Morus nigra*
Mushroom, *Agaricaceae*	Mushroom, *Agaricus bisporus* and *A. campestris*
Mustard, *Cruciferae*	Broccoli, *Brassica oleracea*, var. *italica*
	Brussels sprouts, *Brassica oleracea*, var. *gemmifera*
	Cabbage, *Brassica oleracea*, var. *capitata*
	Cauliflower, *Brassica oleracea*, var. *botrytus*
	Chinese cabbage, *Brassica pekinensis*

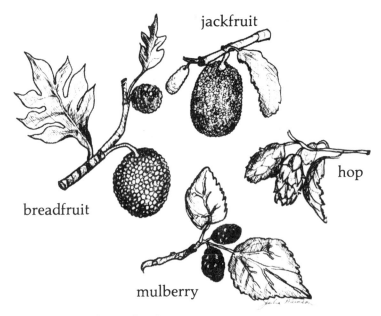

jackfruit

hop

breadfruit

mulberry

Figure 4-9 The mulberry family

Table 4-2 *(continued)*

Family	Plant
	Collards, kale, *Brassica oleracea*, var. *acephala*
	Garden cress, *Lepidium sativum*
	Horseradish, *Roripa armoracia*
	Kohlrabi, *Brassica caulorapa*
	Mustard, *Brassica alba* and *B. nigra*
	Radish, *Raphanus sativus*
	Rapeseed, *Brassica napus*
	Turnip, *Brassica rapa*
	Watercress, *Roripa nasturtium*
	Wintercress, *Barbarea vernapraecox*
Myrtle, *Myrtaceae*	Allspice, *Eugenia pimenta*
	Chilean guava, *Myrtus ugni*
	Clove, *Caryophyllus aromaticus*
	Feijoa, *Feijoa sellowiana*
	Guava, *Psidium guayaba*
	Jambolan, *Eugenia jambolana*

Table 4-2 *(continued)*

Family	Plant
	Myrtle, *Myrtus communis*
	Roseapple, *Eugenia jambos*
	Surninam cherry, *Eugenia latifolia*
Nasturtium, *Tropaeolaceae*	Nasturtium, *Tropaeolum* spp.
Nightshade, *Solanaceae*	Bell (mango) pepper, *Capsicum grossum*
	Cape gooseberry, *Physalis edulis*
	Cayenne pepper, *Capsicum frutescens*
	Currant tomato, *Lyrospericon pipenellifolium*
	Eggplant, *Solanum melongena*
	Ground cherry, *Physalis* spp.
	Paprika, *Capsicum annum*
	Potato (white, Irish), *Solanum tuberosum*
	Tomato, *Lycospericon esculentum*
	Tree tomato, *Cyphomandra betacea*

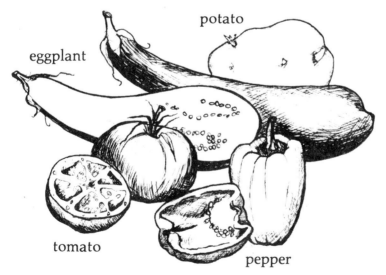

Figure 4-10 The nightshade family

Table 4-2 *(continued)*

Family	Plant
Nutmeg, *Urristicaceae*	Nutmeg, mace, *Myristica fragrans*
Oleaster, *Elaeagnaceae*	Silverberry, *Elaegangnus argentea*
Olive, *Oleaceae*	Jasmine, *Jasminum officinale*
	Manna, *Fraxinus ornus*
	Olive, *Olea europaea*
Orchid, *Orchidaceae*	Salep, *Orchis planifolia*
	Vanilla, *Vanilla* spp.
Palm, *Palmae*	Cabbage palm, *Sabal palmetto*
	Coconut, *Cocus nucifera*
	Cohune nut, *Attalea cohune*
	Date, *Phoenix dactylifera*
	Oil palm, *Elaeis tuinensi*
	Sago palm, *Metroxylon* spp.
Papaya, *Caricaceae*	Papaya, *Carica papaya*
Parsley, *Apiaceae*	Angelica, *Angelica archangelica*
	Anise, *Pimpinella anisum*
	Black cumin, *Nigella sativa*
	Caraway seed, *Carum carvi*
	Carrot, *Daucus carota*
	Celery, celeriac, *Apium graveolens*
	Chervil, *Anthriscus cerefolium*
	Coriander, *Coriandrum sativum*
	Cumin (comino), *Cominum cynimum*
	Dill, *Anethum graveolens*
	Fennel, *Foeniculum vulgare*
	Lovage, *Levisticum officinale*
	Parsley, *Petroselinum hortense*
	Parsnip, *Pastinaca sativa*
	Samphire, *Crithmum martimum*
	Skirret, *Sium sisarum*
	Sweet cicily, *Myrrhis odorata*
	Sweet fennel, *Foeniculum dulce*
Passionflower, *Passifloraceae*	Passion fruit, *Passiflora ilgularis*
Pea, *Leguminosae*	Adzuke (mungo) bean, *Phaseolus mungo*

Table 4-2 *(continued)*

Family	Plant
	Alfalfa, *Medicago sativa*
	Asparagus bean, *Vicia sesquipedalis*
	Balsam of Peru, *Myroxylon pereriae*
	Black-eyed pea, cowpea, *Vigna sinensis*
	Broad (fava) bean, *Vicia faba*
	Carob bean (St. John's bread), *Ceratonia siligua*
	Chickpea (garbanzo), *Cicer arietinum*
	Clover, *Trifolium* spp.
	Common bean (navy, kidney, pinto, string), *Phaseolus vulgaris*
	Fenugreek, *Trigonella faenum-graecum*

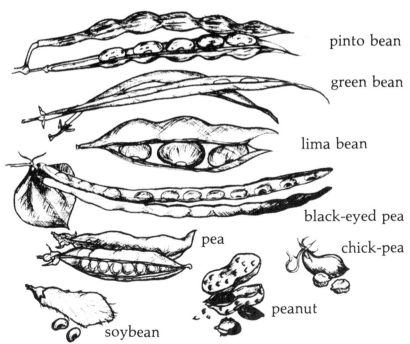

Figure 4-11 The pea family

Table 4-2 *(continued)*

Family	Plant
	Guar, *Cyamopsis tetragonaloba*
	Hyacinth (lablab) bean, *Dioichos lablab*
	Jack bean, *Canavalia ensiformis*
	Lentil, *Lens culanaria*
	Licorice, *Glycyrrhiza glabra*
	Mesquite, *Prosopis glandulosa*
	Pea, *Pisum sativum*
	Peanut, *Arachis hypogaea*
	Pigeonpea, *Dajarium indicus*
	Scarlet runner bean, *Phaseolus coccineus*
	Soybean, *Glycine hispida*
	Tepary bean, *Phaseolus acutifolius*
	Tonka bean, *Coumarouna odorata*
	Tragacanth, *Astragalus gummifer*
	Yambean, *Pachyrhizus* spp.
Pepper, *Piperaceae*	Black (and white) pepper, *Piper niger*
Pine, *Pinaceae*	Juniper, *Juniperus communis*
	Pinyon nut, *Pinus edulis*
Pineapple, *Ananaceae*	Pineapple, *Ananas comosus*
Plum, *Amygdalaceae*	Almond, *Amygdalus communis*
	Apricot, *Prunus armeniaca*
	Cherry, *Prunus avium* and *P. cerasus*
	Peach, nectarine, *Prunus persica*
	Plum, prune, *Prunus* spp.
	Sloe, *Prunus spinosa*
Pokeweed, *Phytolaccaceae*	Pokeweed, *Phytolacca americana*
Pomegranate, *Punicaceae*	Pomegranate, *Punica granatum*
Poppy, *Papaveraceae*	Poppyseed, *Papaver somniferum*
Protea, *Proteaceae*	Macadamia nut, *Macadamia ternifolia*

Table 4-2 *(continued)*

Family	Plant
Purslane, *Portulacaceae*	Purslane, *Portulaca oleracea*
Rose, *Rosaceae*	Black raspberry, *Rubus occidentalis*
	Blackberry, *Rubus* spp.
	Boysenberry, dewberry, logan- berry, *Rubus* spp.
	Burnet, *Sanguisorba minor*
	Cloudberry, *Rubus* spp.
	Dewberry, *Rubus villosus*
	Red raspberry, *Rubus idaeus*
	Rose, *Rosa* spp.
	Strawberry, *Fragaria* spp.
Sac fungi, class *Ascomyceteae*	Morel, *Morchella esculenta*
Sapodilla, *Sapotaceae*	Sapodilla, chicle, *Achras zapota*
	Sapote, *Calocarpus mammosum*
Seaweeds, *Phaeophyceae* and *Rhodophyaceae*	Agar, *Gelidium cartilagineum*
	Bladder weed, *Macrotystis* spp.

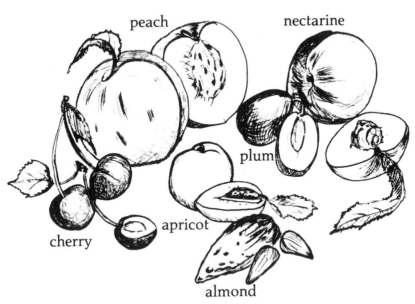

Figure 4-12 The plum family

64

Table 4-2 *(continued)*

Family	Plant
	Carrageen (Irish moss), *Chondrus crispus* and *Gigargina stellata*
	Dulse, *Rhodymenia*
	Laver, *Porphyra* spp.
Senna, *Caesalpinaceae*	Tamarind, *Tamarindus indica.*
Sesame, *Pedaliaceae*	Sesame seed, *Sesamum indicum*
Soapberry, *Sapindaceae*	Ackee, *Blighia sapida*
	Guarana, *Paulinia cupana*
	Litchi, *Litchi chinensis*
	Longan, *Euphora longan*
	Pulasan, *Nephelium mutabile*
	Rambutan, *Nephelium pappaceum*
Spurge, *Euphorbiaceae*	Tapioca, *Manihot manihot*
Star apple, *Sapotaceae*	Star apple, *Chrysophyllum canaito*

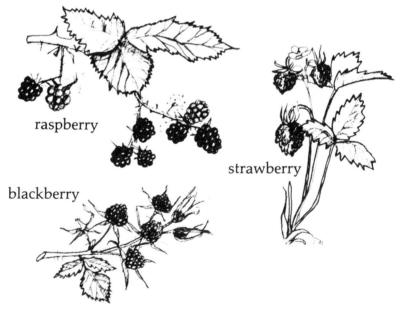

Figure 4-13 The rose family

Table 4-2 *(continued)*

Family	Plant
Sunflower (aster), *Compositae*	Artichoke, *Cynara scolymus*
	Burdock, *Arctium lappa*
	Calendula, *Calendula officinalis*
	Camomile, *Anthemis* spp.
	Cardoon, *Cunara cardunculus*
	Celtuce, *Lactuca sativa,* var. *asparagina*
	Chicory, *Cichorium intybus*
	Costmary, *Chrysanthemum balsamita*
	Dandelion, *Taraxacum taraxacum*
	Endive, escarole, *Cichorium endiva*
	Jerusalem artichoke, *Helianthus tuberosus*
	Lettuce, *Lactuca sativa*
	Rooibusch, *Borbonia cordata*
	Safflower, *Carthanus tinctorius*

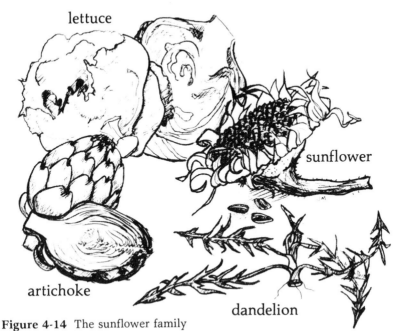

Figure 4-14 The sunflower family

66

Table 4-2 *(continued)*

Family	Plant
	Salsify (oyster plant), *Tragopogon porrifolius*
	Sunflower seed, *Helianthus annuus*
	Tansy, *Tanacetum vulgare*
	Tarragon, *Artemisia drancunculus*
Tea, *Theaceae*	Tea, *Thea sinensis*
Truffle, *Tuberaceae*	Truffle, *Tuber* spp.
Valerian, *Valerianaceae*	Corn salad, *Valerinella olitoris*
Vervain, *Verbenaceae*	Lemon verbena, *Verbena citriodora*
Walnut, *Juglandaceae*	Black walnut, *Juglans nigra*
	Butternut, *Juglans cinerea*
	English walnut, *Juglans regia*
	Hickory nut, *Carya* spp.
	Pecan, *Hicoria pecan*
Water chestnut, *Trapaceae*	Water chestnut, *Trapa natans*
Water lily, *Nymphaceae*	Lotus, *Nelumbo nucifera*
Wood sorrel, *Oxalidaceae*	Bilimbi, *Averhoa bilimbi*
	Gooseberry tree, *Averhoa carambola*
Yam, Dioscoreacea	Yam, *Dioscorea* spp.
Yeast, *Saccharomycetaceae*	Yeast, *Saccharomyces cerevisiae*

Table 4-3
Classification of Animal Foods

Class	Animal
Insect, Insecta	Cochineal, *Dactylopius coccus* (Many insects, locusts being most common, are used as foods in various parts of the world.)
Pelecypoda	Mussel—oyster, clam, cockle, scallop
Gastropoda	Snail—abalone, periwinkle
Cephalopoda	Octopus—squid
Crustacea	Crab—shrimp, lobster, crayfish, prawn
Plagiostomi	Sharks—dogfish

Table 4-3 *(continued)*

Class	Animal
Teleostomi	*Acipenseridae*—sturgeon
	Argentinidae—smelt
	Anguillidae—eel
	Caranigadae—pompano
	Clupedae—herring
	Coryphaenidae—dolphin
	Cyprinadae—carp, chub, dace, roach
	Elopidae—tarpon
	Esocidae—muskellunge, pickerel, pike
	Gadidae—cod, haddock, pollack, whiting
	Histiophoridae—sailfish
	Merlucidae—hake
	Molidae—sunfish
	Mugilidae—mullet
	Percidae—perch
	Pleuronectidae—flounder, halibut
	Pomatonidae—bluefish
	Salmoidae—grayling, salmon, trout, whitefish
	Sciendidae—croaker, drum, redfish, weakfish
	Scombridae—bonito, tuna, mackerel
	Serranidae—grouper, white bass, rock fish
	Siluridae—bullhead, catfish
	Soleidae—sole
	Sparidae—porgy, red snapper
	Spyraenidae—barracuda
	Stolephoridae—anchovy
	Stromateidae—butterfish
	Xyphidae—swordfish
Amphibia	Frog
Reptilia	Turtle, iguana
Aves (birds)	Chicken, duck, turkey, goose, quail, pheasant, dove, egg
Mammalia	Beef, pork, lamb and mutton, cow's and goat's milk, venison, rabbit, squirrel, and many others

Since cross-reactivity in animal foods tends to extend to the class rather than to the family (as is true of plant foods), foods are listed by class. In the case of fish there may be some tendency for cross-reactivity to be confined to a family. For this reason the families of fish are included.

5 • A DISCUSSION
OF INDIVIDUAL FOODS

In this chapter we turn to the most important aspect of food allergy, the foods themselves. To borrow a thought from Alexander Pope, "The proper study of food allergy is foods." We will consider not only the most common offenders but also those that are least allergenic. We are interested not only in what the patient cannot eat but in what he can. This is especially true when we are called on to prescribe a diet for the many patients with multiple food allergy.

When we consider the great number of nourishing and palatable foods available to us, we cannot help but admire the ingenuity and discernment that our remote ancestors showed in choosing those plant and animal products that are both nourishing *and* palatable. From animals they obtained meat, milk, and eggs. From plants they obtained a wide variety of leafy vegetables, root vegetables, fruits, and seeds. They also discovered the edibility of the stems of asparagus and sugarcane, the tubers of potato and water chestnut, the shoots of bamboo and pokeweed, the sprouts of Brussels sprout and beans, the rhizomes of arrowroot and ginger, the bulbs of onion and garlic, the flowers of artichoke and clove, the leaf stalks of celery and rhubarb, the bark of cinnamon and manna, and the sap of maple and birch. They also discovered salt, honey, mushrooms, yeast, the oils of olive and soybean, the starches of tapioca and sago, and all our spices and nuts. They invented cooking and learned how to preserve foods, using salt, vinegar, wine, drying, and freezing. Modern man has his accomplishments, but ancient man gave him his food.

The importance of the physician's learning all he can about the common foods of his part of the world cannot be overemphasized. This is his clear duty. It is also his duty to share this information with his patients. The discussion that follows will aid him in this task. If there is a language barrier between the reader and this book or between him and his patients, Table 5-8, found at the end of this chapter, may be useful. It lists the names of common foods in English, French, Spanish, Italian, and German.

ABALONE

The abalone is a sea snail (marine gastropod) of the Pacific coast, considered by many to be a delicacy. Shell fragments excavated at

Catalina Island reveal that it was used for food as early as four centuries B.C. It seems also to have been nearly exterminated then as it threatens to be today. In the islands of the English Channel a related species known as ormers is also used for food.

ACACIA

The acacias are trees and shrubs important as sources of gum arabic (gum acacia), a food additive used as a stabilizer and thickener. It is considered a valuable food in its own right in parts of Asia and Africa.

ACEROLA

This fruit of the West Indies is closely related to the cherry, with which it could be expected to cross-react. It is a rich source of ascorbic acid.

ACIDS

Many organic acids and one inorganic acid, phosphoric, are naturally present in foods and are especially abundant in fruits. For this reason they are often called "fruit acids," and when used as food additives, are so listed on packages. The most common are citric acid, derived chiefly from citrus fruits but now synthesized, and malic acid, derived chiefly from apple (Latin *malum,* apple). Acids are commonly added to foods to lend tartness and flavor, to permit effective heat processing of canned vegetables without discoloration, and to compensate for insufficient acid in fruits used in making jellies and jams. Acetic acid probably ranks second only to salt as the most commonly used food additive and preservative. In Table 5-1 are listed the sources of acids naturally occurring in foods.

ACKEE (AKEE)

Sturtevant has this to say about ackee: "This small tree is a native of Guinea and was carried to Jamaica by Captain Bligh in 1793. It is much esteemed in the West Indies as a fruit. The fruit is fleshy, of a red color tinged with yellow, about three inches long by two in width of a three-sided form. When ripe, it splits down the middle of each side, disclosing three shining, jet-black seeds, seated upon and partly immersed in a white spongy substance called the aril. This aril is the eatable part."[87] Although it is not certain that the intrepid captain of

Table 5-1
Acids Occurring Naturally in Foods[15,66,132]

Benzoic	Cranberry
Citric	Apricot, artichoke, asparagus, banana, beans, beet, blueberry, broccoli, cabbage, carrot, cauliflower, celery, cranberry, cucumber, currant, fig, grape, grapefruit, lemon, lettuce, okra, onion, orange, parsnip, pea, peach, pear, pineapple, plum, potato, raspberry, rhubarb, spinach, squash, strawberry, tomato
Fumaric	Apple, gooseberry, watermelon
Malic	Apple, apricot, artichoke, asparagus, banana, beans, blackberry, blueberry, broccoli, cabbage, carrot, cauliflower, celery, cherry, cranberry, cucumber, currant, gooseberry, grape, grapefruit, lettuce, okra, onion, parsnip, pea, peach, pear, pineapple, plum, pumpkin, raspberry, rhubarb, spinach, squash, strawberry, tomato, turnip, watermelon
Oxalic	Apricot, blackberry, blueberry, currant, rhubarb, spinach
Quinic	Cranberry, pear
Succinic	Blackberry, cranberry, currant
Tartaric	Apple, artichoke, asparagus, cherry, grape

the *Bounty* brought the ackee to Jamaica, botanists have honored him by giving the plant the scientific name of *Blighia sapida*.

Ackee is known to be poisonous until ripe, causing what is locally known as the vomiting sickness. The toxic principle is a water-soluble hypoglycine.

ACORNS

Throughout Spain, Portugal, and Northern Africa, acorns of certain oaks are commonly used as foods.[168] They are prepared in much the same manner as chestnuts, members of the same botanical family.

ADDITIVES, FOOD

Food additives have always been used to improve the flavor, color, and keeping qualities of meats, fruits, grains, and vegetables. Most spices (which are the most common additives) have been used for thousands of years, many of them being mentioned in the Bible and other ancient writings. Sugar, salt, smoke, wine, and vinegar are other additives of ancient origin.

Now that a small minority of people in the Western world produces food for the great majority, food additives have become essential. It has become fashionable to criticize food manufacturers for using them, even to suggest that we are somehow being "poisoned." All evidence points in the opposite direction: many additives act as nutritional supplements—vitamins, iron, and iodine, for example. Dr. Bernard L. Oser, a former member of the Food Protection Committee of the National Academy of Sciences has said, "Were it not for food additives, baked goods would go stale or mold overnight, salad oils and dressings would separate and turn rancid, table salt would turn hard and lumpy, canned fruits and vegetables would become discolored or mushy, vitamin potencies would deteriorate, beverages and frozen desserts would lack flavor, and wrappings would stick to the contents."[66]

Further discussion of additives and their uses is to be found in this chapter under the headings of Acids, Antioxidants, Colors, Emulsifiers, Flavors, Mold inhibitors, Preservatives, Sequestrants, and Stabilizers and Thickeners.

Table 5-2
Food Additives

Anticaking Agents	*Chemical Preservatives*
Aluminum calcium silicate	Gum guaiac
Calcium silicate	Methylparaben
Magnesium silicate	Potassium bisulfite
Sodium aluminosilicate	Potassium metabisulfite
Sodium calcium	Potassium sorbate
aluminosilicate	Propionic acid
Tricalcium silicate	Propyl gallate
	Propyl paraben
Chemical Preservatives	Sodium ascorbate
	Sodium benzoate
Ascorbic acid	Sodium bisulfite
Ascorbyl palmitate	Sodium metabisulfite
Benzoic acid	Sodium propionate
Butylated hydroxyanisole (BHA)	Sodium sorbate
Butylated hydroxytoluene (BHT)	Sodium sulfite
Calcium ascorbate	Sorbic acid
Calcium propionate	Stannous chloride
Calcium sorbate	Sulfur dioxide
Caprylic acid	Thiodipropionic acid
Dilauryl thiodipropionate	Tocopherols
Erythorbic acid	

Table 5-2 *(continued)*

Emulsifying Agents

Cholic acid
Desoxycholic acid
Diacetyl tartaric acid esters
  of mono- and diglycerides
Glycocholic acid
Mono- and diglycerides
Monosodium phosphate
  derivatives of above
Oxbile extract
Propylene glycol
Taurocholic acid

Nutrients and Dietary Supplements

Alanine
Arginine
Ascorbic acid
Aspartic acid
Biotin
Calcium carbonate
Calcium citrate
Calcium glycerophosphate
Calcium oxide
Calcium pantothenate
Calcium phosphate
Calcium pyrophosphate
Calcium sulfate
Carotene
Choline bitartrate
Choline chloride
Copper gluconate
Cuprous iodide
Cysteine
Cystine
Ferric phosphate
Ferric pyrophosphate
Ferric sodium pyrophosphate
Ferrous gluconate
Ferrous lactate
Ferrous sulfate
Glycine
Histidine
Inositol
Iron, reduced
Isoleucine

Nutrients and Dietary Supplements

Leucine
Linoleic acid
Lysine
Magnesium oxide
Magnesium phosphate
Magnesium sulfate
Manganese chloride
Manganese citrate
Manganese gluconate
Manganese glycerophosphate
Manganese hypophosphite
Manganese sulfate
Manganous oxide
Mannitol
Methionine
Methionine hydroxy analogue
Niacin
Niacinamide
D-pantothenyl alcohol
Phenylalanine
Potassium chloride
Potassium glycerophosphate
Potassium iodide
Proline
Pyridoxine hydrochloride
Riboflavin
Riboflavin-5-phosphate
Serine
Sodium pantothenate
Sodium phosphate
Sorbitol
Thiamine hydrochloride
Thiamine mononitrate
Threonine
Tocopherols
Tocopherol acetate
Tryptophane
Tyrosine
Valine
Vitamin A
Vitamin A acetate
Vitamin A palmitate
Vitamin B_{12}
Vitamin D_2
Vitamin D_3

74

Table 5-2 *(continued)*

Nutrients and Dietary Supplements

Zinc chloride
Zinc gluconate
Zinc oxide
Zinc stearate
Zinc sulfate

Sequestrants

Calcium acetate
Calcium chloride
Calcium citrate
Calcium diacetate
Calcium gluconate
Calcium hexametaphosphate
Calcium phosphate, monobasic
Calcium phytate
Citric acid
Dipotassium phosphate
Disodium phosphate
Isopropyl citrate
Monoisopropyl citrate
Potassium citrate
Sodium acid phosphate
Sodium citrate
Sodium diacetate
Sodium gluconate
Sodium hexametaphosphate
Sodium metaphosphate
Sodium phosphate
Sodium potassium tartrate
Sodium pyrophosphate
Sodium pyrophosphate, tetra
Sodium tartrate
Sodium thiosulfate
Sodium tripolyphosphate
Stearyl citrate
Tartaric acid

Stabilizers

Acacia (gum arabic)
Agar-agar
Ammonium alginate
Calcium alginate
Carob bean gum

Stabilizers

Chondrus extract
Ghatti gum
Guar gum
Potassium alginate
Sodium alginate
Sterculia (or karaya) gum
Tragacanth

Miscellaneous Additives

Acetic acid
Adipic acid
Aluminum ammonium sulfate
Aluminum potassium sulfate
Aluminum sodium sulfate
Aluminum sulfate
Ammonium bicarbonate
Ammonium carbonate
Ammonium hydroxide
Ammonium phosphate
Ammonium sulfate
Beeswax
Bentonite
Butane
Caffeine
Calcium carbonate
Calcium chloride
Calcium citrate
Calcium gluconate
Calcium hydroxide
Calcium lactate
Calcium oxide
Calcium phosphate
Caramel
Carbon dioxide
Carnauba wax
Citric acid
Dextrans
Ethyl formate
Glutamic acid
Glutamic acid hydrochloride
Glycerin
Glyceryl monostearate
Helium
Hydrochloric acid

Table 5-2 *(continued)*

Miscellaneous Additives	*Miscellaneous Additives*
Hydrogen peroxide	Sodium sesquicarbonate
Lactic acid	Sodium tripolyphosphate
Lecithin	Succinic acid
Magnesium carbonate	Sulfuric acid
Magnesium hydroxide	Tartaric acid
Magnesium oxide	Triacetin
Magnesium stearate	Triethylcitrate
Malic acid	
Methylcellulose	*Synthetic Flavoring Substances*
Monoammonium glutamate	
Monopotassium glutamate	Acetaldehyde
Nitrogen	Acetoin
Nitrous oxide	Aconitic acid
Papain	Anethole
Phosphoric acid	Benzaldehyde
Potassium acid tartrate	n-butyric acid
Potassium bicarbonate	d- or l-carvone
Potassium carbonate	Cinnamaldehyde
Potassium citrate	Citral
Potassium hydroxide	Decanal
Potassium sulfate	Diacetyl
Propane	Ethyl acetate
Propylene glycol	Ethyl butyrate
Rennet	Ethyl vanillin
Silica aerogel	Eugenol
Sodium acetate	Geraniol
Sodium acid pyrophosphate	Geranyl acetate
Sodium aluminum phosphate	Glycerol tributyrate
Sodium bicarbonate	Limonene
Sodium carbonate	Linalool
Sodium carboxymethylcellulose	Linalyl acetate
Sodium caseinate	l-malic acid
Sodium citrate	Methyl anthranilate
Sodium hydroxide	3-Methyl-3-phenyl glycidic
Sodium pectinate	acid ethyl ester
Sodium phosphate	Piperonal
Sodium potassium tartrate	Vanillin

Group of additives included in the U.S. Food and Drug Administration's list of additives "generally recognized as safe" is given, except for large groups of natural flavors and oils. To be on this list an additive must have been in use before 1958 and have met certain specifications of safety. Additives brought into use since 1958 must be approved individually. Occasionally substances are removed from the list by the FDA in the light of new evidence; recent examples are the cyclamate sweeteners and saccharin.

ADULTERANTS

National food and drug laws (and those who have the thankless task of enforcing them) have had remarkable success in suppressing the age-old merchandizing practice of palming off inferior, even toxic, substitutes as good food. As recently as 1887, the *Journal of the American Medical Association* reported:

> A most plausible currant jelly, sold until a year ago by nearly every grocer and fruiterer, was made as follows: Dried apples, glucose, water, arsenical fuchsine (a red aniline pigment), tartaric acid, and glue. This mixture was boiled and strained, and sufficient salicylic acid added to keep it from spoiling in hot weather. There are very few of the fruit jellies sold now which are not frauds, though many of them are not dangerous to health. The apple does duty for almost every fruit, the other ingredients being glucose, water, color, flavors, and gelatine.

> Coffee and tea are adulterated. Almost all green teas are artificially colored; usually with Prussian blue, turmeric, or soapstone. . . . Vermicelli is sometimes colored with chromate of lead instead of eggs or saffron. The notorious "egg powder" is a new name of chrome yellow or lead chromate.[56]

It is an irony of history that medical groups, health departments, and other promoters of pure foods are attacked by food faddists for an alleged conspiracy with manufacturers to make the modern diet deficient or even harmful. Speaking from the point of view of a layman, Klaw has pointed out the "profound distrust of the medical establishment" that has always existed in America.[110] As to the self-appointed food experts, Dr. Ruth Leverton of the Department of Agriculture comments, "We find it hard to understand how so many people could so rapidly have become experts in the field without benefit of training—and with their only experience having been that of eating."[112]

AGAR (AGAR-AGAR)

Familiar to medical students as the base of bacterial culture media, agar is also used as a food. It consists of a complex mixture of polysaccharides obtained from various seaweeds. It is used in food manufacture as a thickening agent in candies, jellies, and salad dressings.

ALLSPICE

This widely used spice is so called because its flavor and aroma resemble that of a mixture of the common spices, especially cinnamon, nutmeg, and clove. Its source is the allspice or pimento tree, and it is sometimes known as the pimento. It is unrelated to the pimiento pepper of the nightshade family.

ALMOND

The almond is a fruit of the plum family whose seed is one of our most popular nuts. It is a close relative of the peach, with which it sometimes hybridizes. Allergy to almond has no connection with allergy to nuts of other families. It may cross-react, at least to some extent, with other members of the plum family.

ANGELICA

The roots and fruits of this member of the parsley family are used in flavoring liqueurs and candies, pastries, and Italian dishes. It is the flavoring agent in anisette.

ANNATTO

The seeds of the annatto tree contain a yellow-red pigment used in coloring butter and cheeses. It has been largely replaced by beta-carotene, a precursor of vitamin A.

ANTIOXIDANTS

We have all noticed that apples, peaches, and potatoes turn brown soon after they are sliced and exposed to the air; we also know how easily oils and fats become rancid. These reactions are caused by oxidation, a serious problem to the food processor. Agents used to prevent this include ascorbic acid, vitamin E, erythordic acid, sodium sulfite, sulfur dioxide, BHA (butylated hydroxyanisole), BHT (butylated hydroxytoluene), and propyl gallate. (See BHA/BHT and Sulfites.)

APPLE

Perhaps no fruit is so widely used or so variable in type as the apple. It is available as the fresh fruit and as a constituent of pastries (pies, dumplings, etc), cider (apple juice), hard cider, brandy, and apple cider vinegar. It is the chief source of pectin used in the preparation of jellies. Apple is a fairly common allergen, especially as a cause of gastrointestinal allergy and aphthous stomatitis. Strange to say, many patients have trouble only with the peeling.

Johnstone has told of how the father of an English physician, aged 65, was accidentally cured of eczema while in the hospital for cataract surgery:

> His love for apples was great and he took a large supply with him, but his pride and independence were even greater. In those days, after an operation for cataract, it was a strict rule that the patient should move as little as possible. When he wasn't allowed to reach for his apples, he refused to ask the nurse to hand one to him. During the rest of the time in bed he discovered a remarkable improvement in his eczematous condition, which had caused him much inconvenience over the past 10 years. Thereafter, by avoiding raw or cooked apples, he remained free of eczema until his death at 80 years of age.[100]

APRICOT

The apricot is closely related to the peach botanically but not allergenically.

ARROWROOT

The common arrowroot of commerce is West Indian arrowroot, which is derived from the rhizomes or *Maranta* app. For patients on a wheat-free diet, it is useful as a thickening agent for home preparation of gravies, soups, stews, and cream sauces.

Other starches known as arrowroot are Florida arrowroot, from rhizomes of a cycad, *Zamia florida,* the Seminole bread plant; Queensland arrowroot, from the rhizomes of a canna, *Canna edulis;* and East India arrowroot, from the rhizomes of a member of the ginger family, *Curcuma angustifolia.*[115]

ARTICHOKE, GLOBE

Also called the common, green, Italian, or true artichoke, the globe artichoke is one of our most delicious vegetables. The part used for food is the fleshy base of the immature flower buds and bracts ("leaves"). It occasionally is allergenic. (See also Jerusalem artichoke.)

ASPARAGUS

The chlorophyl-containing shoots of this plant act as leaves. Asparagus is one of our most popular vegetables; unfortunately, it has become expensive. It is, however, easily grown and should be in every home garden in the parts of the country where it thrives. It occasionally cross-reacts with onion and garlic as they are all members of the same botanical family. In 1898 Deschamps reported the case of a chef who could eat asparagus but not endure its odor:

> From the first he found that while trimming asparagus in the kitchen, violent sneezing, coryza, and running in the eyes set in. Within half an hour dyspnea followed with cough and expectoration. All these symptoms used to vanish within an hour or two.[46]

AVOCADO

The avocado, formerly known as the alligator pear, is a native of Mexico. The Spanish name *aquacate* is derived from the Nahuatl *ahuacatl,* testicle. Avocado is related to cinnamon and bay leaf and may cross-react with them. One of my patients, a young man, reports that he becomes hoarse if he eats one avocado and loses his voice entirely if he eats two. He has a similar reaction to cinnamon, a member of the same botanical family.

BAKING POWDER

The usual ingredients of commercial baking powder are soda, cream of tartar (potassium acid tartrate), tartaric acid, and either sodium aluminum sulfate or monocalcium phosphate. For the purpose of slowing down the leavening reaction that produces carbon dioxide, either wheat flour or corn starch is added.

BALM

The leaves and stems of balm (especially lemon balm) are used in flavoring wines and tea.

BAMBOO

Although they are treelike and may reach a height of 120 feet, bamboos are grasses and are closely related to such common food plants as corn and wheat. In the Western world their use as a food is limited to the familiar bamboo shoots of Chinese dishes. Like other grasses, the bamboos have stems containing sugar, and a syrup is made from them. The fruits of some species are said to have a flavor resembling corn on the cob.

BANANA

The banana is one of our most nutritious and delicious fruits. It is a fairly common food allergen. Some people, allergic or otherwise, find that it causes burning of the tongue and gastric distress, especially when not fully ripe. This does not appear to be an allergic reaction.

Plantain, a large variety of banana, is widely used in many parts of the world as a cooked vegetable. It is now appearing in American markets.

BARLEY

This grain is highly adaptable to various climates and soils and is therefore a useful food in areas where other grains do not thrive. It is known to have been cultivated as early as 5,000 years ago. It is not well adapted to baking because of its low content of gluten and its inferior flavor. Its widest use is in the production of malt. (See also Beer.)

Because barley is closely related allergenically to wheat and rice, it is not an acceptable substitute for either.

BASIL

One of the many members of the mint family, basil is used in tomato pastes, soups, stews, and in vegetable dishes in general. It is present in chartreuse and other liqueurs.

BAY LEAF

This herb, a member of the laurel family, is commonly used in meat dishes. It seems to cross-react completely with cinnamon.

BEAN

The word bean was for many centuries limited to the broad or fava bean of Europe. It is well known as a precipitating factor in favism. (See Chapter 2.)

When the Europeans came to the Western Hemisphere, they were introduced to several related legumes, including lima beans and the many varieties of the common bean. Throughout the years many other types of beans have been discovered, and there are at least 30 species in use in various parts of the world. Among these are mung bean (golden or green gram), carob bean, soybean, cowpea, scarlet runner bean (popular in England), tepary (Texas) bean, urd (black gram), adjuki bean, jack bean, hyacanth (lablab) bean, yambean, asparagus bean, and moth bean.

The common bean, *Phaseolus vulgaris*, has these varieties: navy bean, red bean, kidney bean, great northern bean, black bean, pinto bean, and pea bean. Many of its varieties are used for the production of green beans, also known as French, snap, or string beans. The dry, or mature, beans are most allergenic, but an occasional patient is especially sensitive to green beans. This indicates a reaction to the jelly-like part of the fruit rather than the immature seed.

BEEF

In the Western world beef is the most widely consumed meat. It is a potent allergen but not a common offender. The meat of younger cattle, veal and baby beef, do not seem to differ in allergenicity from ordinary beef. Ground beef is classified as follows: hamburger: 25% to 30% fat; ground chuck: 15% to 20% fat; lean chuck: 10% to 15% fat. In my experience beef-sensitive patients are invariably allergic to milk.

Since they are not popular, it is difficult to say if such organs and glands of cattle as liver, thymus, kidney, and pancreas cross-react with beef. But it is likely they do since it is unusual for one part of an organism not to cross-react with other parts.

Doubt has been expressed as to the safety of the administration of diethylstilbestrol to beef cattle. According to Jukes, traces may sometimes be detected in livers but not in muscle meat.[104]

BEER

Beer is by far the world's most popular alcoholic beverage and the most likely to cause an allergic reaction, but it is not always apparent which constituents of beer cause trouble. In some cases it appears to be the yeast, and this is to be expected in mold-sensitive patients. It may be the alcohol itself, and in this case, of course, the patient must avoid all alcoholic drinks. Frequently it is the corn used in most American beers that is at fault. There are other grains in beer, but I have not been able to implicate them. I know of no case where hops have been the cause of trouble.

The brewing of beer begins with malt, a product of the enzymes of grain (usually barley), acting on the starches of the various grains employed to produce sugar. The sugar is then coverted to alcohol by

82

selected strains of yeast, the familiar brewer's yeast. Hops are added for flavor.

BEET

Both the leaves and roots of the garden beet are nourishing and delicious foods, especially when fresh from the garden. They rarely cause allergic symptoms. Sugar beets are an important source of sugar, which, like other disaccharides (and monosaccharides), is nonallergenic.

BHA/BHT

Two closely related antioxidants, BHA (butylated hydroxyanisole) and BHT (butylated hydroxytoluene) have been shown to be capable of causing such symptoms as rhinitis, wheezing, somnolence, and headache. Challenge doses varied from 125 mg to 250 mg.[64]

BLACK PEPPER

This is the world's most popular spice, the fruit of a vine of Southeast Asia. White pepper is the same fruit with the hull removed. Either black or white pepper is used in almost all highly spiced foods, especially in meats, sauces, pickles, salads, and egg dishes. According to Jones:

> The Western Hemisphere might not have been discovered until a much later date had Columbus not been able to convince financial backers of the possibility of finding pepper and other spices....Magellan's expedition circled the globe in search of spices, and although the great mariner lost his life and all his ships but one foundered, the pepper in the hold of the surviving vessel more than paid for the loss of the ships.[102]

BLACKBERRY

This is one of many fruits of the rose family. It is not a berry but a conglomerate fruit much more closely related to apple and peach than to such true berries as gooseberry, blueberry, and tomato. Varieties of blackberry are loganberry and boysenberry. (See also Raspberry, Strawberry.)

BLUEBERRY

Blueberries of various kinds are in the same genus as huckleberry and bilberry. They are rarely, if ever, allergenic.

BORAGE

The leaves of this plant are used in salads. Their flavor is said to resemble that of the cucumber.

BRAZIL NUT

The Brazil nut, as is true of many foods known as nuts, is actually a seed. Except for its close relative the exotic paradise nut, it is unrelated to all other foods.

Allergy to Brazil nut is not especially common but it is invariably severe. Golbert et al reported a patient so sensitive that he had a constitutional reaction to a scratch test, a rare occurrence.[75]

BREADFRUIT

This fruit, along with the related breadnut, is a staple food of the South Pacific. It may be boiled, baked, or fried.

BROCCOLI

Certain foods, because of their low allergenicity, good flavor, and nutritional value, are useful in feeding highly allergic patients. Broccoli is such a food.

BRUSSELS SPROUTS

Like broccoli, a closely related plant, Brussels sprouts are useful in providing compatible foods for many patients with multiple food allergy.

BUCKWHEAT

There are many kinds of wheat, but buckwheat is not one of them. It belongs to an entirely different botanical family whose only other common food plant is rhubarb. It is therefore useful as a substitute for wheat and the other small grains (rice, barley, oats, rye). It can itself occasionally cause severe reactions, much more severe than those caused by wheat and its relatives.[83,169]

Buckwheat is available as flour for making pancakes and waffles, and as groats (kasha) for use in soups and other dishes. A surprising finding is that it is an unusually valuable source of essential amino acids. According to the studies of Pomeranz and Robbins,'' . . . chemical assays indicate that buckwheat has a better balance and better potential than cereal grains of supplementing foods which are low in lysine.''[147] In similar studies, Shure states, ''The proteins in buckwheat at an 8% level of protein intake are the best known source of high biological value in the plant kingdom, having 92.3% of the value of nonfat milk solids and 81.4% of dried whole eggs.''[189] Since buckwheat thrives under conditions unacceptable for the cereal grains it is obvious that its production should be encouraged where such conditions prevail.

CABBAGE

Few, if any, vegetables are more widely used than this member of the mustard family. Its most common uses are in slaw, as boiled cabbage, and as sauerkraut. It is also remarkable in having so many varieties, shapes, and colors. One delicious variety is Chinese (celery) cabbage. Nonheading varieties, such as kale and collards, are popular in many parts of the world.

CACTUS

In certain desert areas, cacti are important food sources. The pitaya and prickly pear of our own Southwest and Mexico are examples.

CAFFEINE

Among the plants known to contain caffeine are coffee, tea, cola nut, chocolate, maté, and guarana. It is added to soft drinks, principally cola drinks. Although caffeine does not appear to be a direct cause of allergic manifestations, many allergic patients, especially if they have multiple sensitizations, find that caffeine causes restlessness, tremor, tachycardia, and insomnia.

Coffee is said to contain about 15 to 20 mg of caffeine per ounce, tea about 8 mg per ounce, and cola drinks from 3 to 4 mg per ounce. A chocolate bar may contain from 50 to 75 mg.[6] Caffeine is found in many drug preparations. Cafergot, for example, contains 100 mg per tablet. The APC (aspirin-phenacetin-caffeine) tablet so commonly used in World War II contains 30 mg.

CALENDULA

The dried flower heads of this plant, also known as pot marigold, are used as flavorings for soups and stews.

CANTALOUPE

Cantaloupe, muskmelon, and honeydew melon (the terms are often and incorrectly used interchangeably) are used as breakfast fruits and in salads. As is true of melons in general, cantaloupe is not easily digested by many people and, for some reason, often makes the symptoms of ragweed hay fever worse.

CAPE GOOSEBERRY

Most fruits of the nightshade family, such as tomatoes, eggplant, and peppers, are eaten as vegetables; cape gooseberry is eaten as a fruit. In Hawaii it is known as poha.

CAPERS

As a gourmet flavoring, the flowering heads are available in pickled form. I have recently seen a patient severely allergic to capers.

CARAWAY SEEDS

These seeds add agreeable flavor to cheeses, cakes, cookies, rolls, breads, crackers, sauerkraut, pickles, and alcoholic drinks. It is the principal flavoring agent in rye bread.

CARBONATED DRINKS

The soft drinks so popular in the United States are usually sweetened with sugar, colored with caramel or coal tar dyes, and flavored with natural and synthetic flavors. Ginger ale contains citrus oils, fruit juices, caramel, organic acids, and ginger. Root beer may contain any combination of many ingredients, including sarsaparilla, licorice, anise, wintergreen, sassafras, hops, ginger, coriander, clove, dandelion root, wild cherry bark, althea, vanilla, angelica, allspice, yellow dock, caramel, and phosphoric acid. The formulas of cola drinks are secret (as are those of many other soft drinks), but they generally contain cola extract, sugar, vanilla, caffeine, and caramel. There is a recent tendency to use corn syrup in these products.

CARDAMOM

Almost as often spelled cardamon, the seeds of several species of this member of the ginger family supply not only a useful spice but a flavoring used to cover the unpleasant taste of medications. Like its relatives ginger and turmeric, it rarely acts as an allergen.

CARDOON

This plant is a thistle of the same genus as globe artichoke. The leaves are cooked as greens, and the leaf stalks are cooked in the same way as asparagus.

CAROB BEAN (ST. JOHN'S BREAD, LOCUST)

Because of a fancied resemblance of its pods to the insect, the name locust has been given to the pod of this bean. Occidentals, not knowing that the insect itself was a common food in Biblical times, reasoned that when the Scruptures read, "And his meat was locusts and wild honey," it must have been the bean and not the insect that was meant. Hence the name St. John's bread. Since carob beans were also given to swine, it is reasoned that the husks that the Prodigal Son would fain eat were of the same origin.

The sweet pulp of the carob bean is the edible portion, as it is of the pods of the common American locust tree (thorny locust) and mesquite. It is also much of what we enjoy when we eat green beans and snow peas. Dried carob bean pulp is used in the manufacture of chocolate substitutes; such products are to be found in all health food stores.

CARRAGEEN

A coastal Irish village gives its name to this seaweed, also called Irish moss. The active ingredient, carrageenin, is now obtained chiefly from the eastern coast of Canada. It is used as a stabilizer, thickening agent, and emulsifier.

CARROT

Many vegetables and fruits are allergenic when raw but not when cooked. This is usually true of carrot. Carrot is closely related to celery and a number of spices, the most important being dill, coriander, anise, cumin (comino), celery seed, and caraway seed.

CASHEW

The cashew tree produces both a fruit and a nut. (Technically, the "fruit" is the receptacle and the "nut" the ovary). The fresh fruit commonly causes a dermatitis similar to that caused by its relatives, poison ivy, poison oak, and mango. However, the responsible oleoresin is not present in commercial cashew nuts.

CASSAVA

(See Tapioca.)

CASSIA

The bark of the cassia tree produces a spice closely related botanically and in flavor to true cinnamon. In fact, almost all the "cinnamon" sold in the United States is derived from this plant.

CAULIFLOWER

This close relative of cabbage is grown for its edible flower stalks.

CELERY

Like rhubarb, celery represents the stalks of leaves. A related plant, celeriac, is cultivated for its edible root.

CELTUCE

The hybrid name of this vegetable tells us that it resembles celery, but it is actually a variety of lettuce.

CERIMAN

This fruit of a climbing tropical plant is said to have a flavor resembling a blend of banana, strawberry, and pineapple.

CHAYOTE

This is the fruit of a tropical vine. Other names are mirliton, custard marrow, and choco. It also yields a large tuber, which is used in the same way as yam.

CHEESE

The milk of any herbiverous animal can be used to make cheese, but cow's milk is the one most commonly used. The essential steps in cheese production are fermentation, clotting, and ripening. The process of fermentation depends on lactic acid organisms, chiefly *Streptococcus lactis* and *S. cremoris*. Fermentation leads to souring, the enzymes of the lactic acid organisms breaking lactose down to lactic, acetic, and proprionic acids. Clotting occurs with the addition to the sour milk of rennet, an enzyme obtained from the calf's stomach. With clotting, the curd is formed, and the whey is squeezed out, leaving casein and fats. The curd is allowed to ripen, a process which involves the breaking down of both the casein and fats. Cottage cheese is a soft unripened cheese made from skim milk. The blue cheeses contain a mold, *Penicillium camemberti,* and Roquefort cheese contains *P. roqueforti.* Since all species of *Penicillium* contain penicillin, penicillin-sensitive patients should avoid these cheeses. Occasionally patients sensitive to air-borne molds, such as *Alternaria* and *Cladosporium,* have symptoms from the odor of blue cheeses.

As far as has been determined, patients sensitive to milk tend to be allergic to all its proteins. Although cheeses contain mostly casein, and that in broken-down form, milk-sensitive patients generally must avoid them. On a practical basis, however, small amounts can be eaten by most patients, especially if they do not make it a regular practice.

CHERIMOYA

This fruit is one of four tropical fruits of the custard apple family. It is said to have a delicately sweet, acidulous flavor.

CHERRY

Among the many species of cherry, the most widely used are the sweet cherry, *Prunus avium,* and the sour cherry, *Prunus cerasus.* Although the cherry is in the same genus with plum and in the same family as almond, peach, and apricot, it cross-reacts with them very little.

CHERVIL

Two types of this plant are used as foods: one is the salad chervil; the other, the turnip-rooted chervil.

CHESTNUT

One of the saddest stories in the history of botany is how a fungus spread from a Japanese chestnut in the New York Botanical Gardens, rapidly and completely destroying our native chestnut. This occurred in 1904, and attempts to reintroduce it in a fungus-resistant form are achieving questionable success. The story is similar to that of the current Dutch elm blight.

The chestnuts that are found in the United States are imported from Europe. They are a potential source of variety and nutrition in the diet of patients with multiple food allergy. They are commonly eaten roasted and are used to some extent in dressing for poultry. Also available is the purée of chestnut; recipes for its use can be found in gourmet cookbooks.

CHEWING GUM

Originally made entirely from chicle, chewing gum base now may contain the following materials: chicle, natural and artificial rubber, jelutong, paraffin, petroleum wax, polyethylene polysorbate, polyvinyl acetate, rosins, lanolin, rice bran wax, sterates, butylated hydrooxyanisole, hydrooxytoluene, propyl gallate, and sodium sulfide. Flavoring agents include mint, wintergreen, and cinnamon. The usual sweetening agent is corn syrup. Most chewing gum contains artificial food colors or lakes.[106]

I have seen one case in which artificial rubber in chewing gum was the obvious cause of cheilitis and perioral eczema. The patient, a woman in her forties, had a history of severe contact dermatitis from artificial rubber in shoes, elastic, and sponge rubber powder puffs. On one occasion she asked one of her youngsters if she could try some of his bubble gum. The reaction on her lips and perioral skin was severe.

Kleinman reported two cases of allergy to chicle. The most dramatic was that of a 16-year-old boy who complained that every time he chewed gum he had fits of sneezing, itching and swelling of the eyes, and spasmodic coughing. These symptoms came on about half an hour after he began chewing gum and lasted about two hours. He was tested intradermally with concentrated chicle extract. Within three minutes he began to sneeze and develop severe eye congestion and redness. Within 15 minutes he went into an attack of asthma, which required epinephrine for relief.[111]

CHICKEN

Reactions to the meats of birds, like those to meats of mammals, are not especially common, but when they occur they are inclined to be severe. In 1888, 18 years before the term allergy was coined, we find this comment by a British physician:

> My first lesson in this way was taken early in my practice by observing the prompt cure of a stubborn and annoying supra-orbital neuralgia, one which had resisted my efforts for months, and which promptly yielded after a visit of my patient to a Chinese physician, who advised the discontinuance of poultry from the diet list.

And yet today, almost a century later, the possibility that food may be a cause of headache is generally ignored!

Even more important and widely used than the meat of chicken is its egg (q.v.). Whether there is any cross-reaction between chicken meat and chicken egg is doubtful. However, exquisitely egg-sensitive patients may have trouble with the meat of *hens,* a phenomenon that seems to depend on the presence of circulating egg proteins in the hen.

Other birds used as foods are doves, duck, goose, grouse, Guinea fowl, ostrich, partridge, peafowl, pheasant, plover, prairie chicken, ptarmigan, quail, snipe, turkey, and woodcock. Since chicken allergy is uncommon and turkey is eaten only occasionally I am not sure whether there is cross-reactivity between the two. If there is, of course, the patient will soon discover it.

CHICORY

Growing along the roadsides of America is a persistent weed with beautiful blue flowering heads somewhat resembling the aster. This is chicory, a close relative of the dandelion. And, like the dandelion, its young and tender leaves make excellent greens. But its more widely used part is the root, which is dried and ground and roasted with coffee. Since it adds flavor, it is not considered an adulterant.

CHILI POWDER

In his fascinating book, *A Treasury of Spices,* Jones lists the constituents of chili powder as follows:

> A blend of spices, usually chili pepper, cumin seed, and oregano. Other spices are often added today in making the blend. The use of chili peppers and oregano in combination has been traced back to the Aztecs. The pre-mixed blend we call chili powder, however, is an American innovation, having originated in our own Southwest during the nineteenth century. Although it is a basic seasoning of chili con carne and all Mexican-type dishes, chili powder is also excellent in eggs, omelettes, etc.[102]

Other ingredients of chili are pinto beans *(frijoles),* tomato, and beef, plus such spices as paprika, garlic, clove, mustard, corn syrup, and cinnamon. Most commercial chili contains wheat flour.

CHIVES

Resembling the leaves of the related onion, chives are widely used in salads, cheeses, soups, omelets, and potato chip dips. They are less prone than onions to cause indigestion or to leave a bad taste in the mouth.

CHOCOLATE

Chocolate and cola (with which chocolate cross-reacts closely, if not completely) are the two most common food-plant allergens. The history of chocolate was told in 1887 by the great physician-naturalist, E. Lewis Sturtevant:

> When Cortez was entertained at the court of the Aztec Emperor, Montezuma, he was treated to a sweet preparation of the cocoa, called *chocollatl,* flavored with vanilla and other aromatic spices. Cocoa (cacao) was carried to Spain from Mexico, and the Spaniards kept the cacao secret for many years, selling it very profitably as chocolate to the wealthy and luxurious classes of Europe. Chocolate reached France, however, only in 1661 and did not reach Britain until a few years later. It is now more largely consumed in Spain than elsewhere in Europe. The European consumption of chocolate is estimated at quite 40 million pounds. In the United States, the imports in 1880 were over 7 million pounds.

> Cacao was cultivated by the nations of Central America before the arrival of Europeans. The Nahua Nations used the nibs, or grains, as

circulating medium instead of money. Stephens states that the nuts are still used in Yucatan as currency, as of old, by the Indians. After maize, says Landa, cacao was perhaps the crop to which the most attention was paid.[87]

Chocolate and cola are capable of causing any manifestation of food allergy but are especially common causes of common and classic migraine. Chocolate is used in all sorts of sweets and desserts, such as candies, cakes, pies, rolls, drinks, and ice cream. The physician need spend little time identifying chocolate as an allergen in adults, since the patient usually has identified it long before he presents himself for treatment. It is more easily overlooked in children. Cocoa is the term given to de-fatted chocolate. Milk chocolate, the type used in candies, contains 20 percent milk. (See also Caffeine, Cola.)

CINNAMON

True cinnamon has been replaced in this country almost entirely by the related cassia. True cinnamon is *Cinnamomum zeylanicum,* and cassia is *Cinnamomum cassia.* In any case, the spice we call cinnamon is a common allergen, the most common of the spice allergens. It is a delicious spice and is to be found in almost any food that is at once sweet and spicy, such as apple dishes, pumpkin pie, cakes, cookies, and tomato catsup.

If patients find that such dishes as apple pie, dumplings, and sauce cause symptoms, the most likely cause is cinnamon, a spice they regularly contain.

CITRON

This minor member of the citrus family is used in candied form in fruit cakes, mincemeat, candies, and various highly seasoned baked goods.

CITRUS FLAVORS

Citric acid is found in a wide variety of fruits, but is especially rich in the citrus fruits (orange, lemon, grapefruit, etc) and pineapple. The chief commercial source is lemon peel. Also obtained from citrus fruits are essential oils; they add greatly to the flavor of such products as carbonated drinks and gelatine desserts. Citric acid and citrus oils may cause minor allergic symptoms.

CLAM

(See Mollusks.)

CLOVE

The unopened flower buds of clove resemble old-fashioned carpenter's nails. It is therefore appropriate that the word clove be derived from the French *clau*, nail. Clove is among the least likely of the spices to cause allergy.

COCHINEAL

This is perhaps the only food product of insect origin that is universally acceptable. The female of the insect *Dactylus coccus*, attaches to small cacti, sucking the sap. When ready for market, the insects are brushed off into a basket and then baked. The scarlet dye that is produced is used in coloring foods and beverages. Because of its expense, its use is limited.

COCONUT

The nut of the coconut palm is the source of the world's most common edible oil. The shredded meat is used in cookies, candies, and cakes.

A great gourmet dish is the salad made from shoots of the terminal bud. However, this "palm cabbage" is very expensive since its removal kills the tree. Its flavor much resembles celery and is delicious. While I was serving in the South Pacific, several trees were felled to make room for a building. With the help of salt, pepper, and vinegar from the galley, and mineral oil from the sick bay, our Filipino mess cooks favored us with this great treat.

COFFEE

Coffee, next to water the most popular drink in the world, is an infusion of the seeds of various small trees of the genus *Caffea*. It is valued for its content of caffeine and for its aroma. The aroma comes chiefly from an essential oil, caffeol. Coffee is prepared in various ways from the ground "beans" or from "instant" soluble powder. No food (if coffee is a food) has so many complexities as to cultivation, variety, blending, and brewing.

It is remarkable how many people have a feeling that coffee is "bad" for them. Everyone has observed a scene like this: The coffee drinker, having finished his meal, settles back in his chair and eyes his cup. Offered another cup, he replies, "I shouldn't. But just a little."

Actually, the coffee habit does not appear to be as hazardous to health as cigarette addiction. It is true that it may cause indigestion, insomnia, breath odor, and tremor, but attempts to link it to cancer and cardiovascular disease are not convincing.

With the notable exception of headache, coffee rarely causes true allergic manifestations. It is worthy of note, however, that highly allergic people seldom tolerate it, complaining chiefly of indigestion and general nervousness.

Coffee contains a number of active chemicals, most of which no food chemist would dare use as additives. Some of those listed by Benarde are: acetaldehyde, acetic acid, acetone, ammonia, cresols, ethyl alcohol, eugenol, formic acid, furfural, guiacol, hydrogen sulfide, hydro-quinone, methyl alcohol, phenol, pyridine, and resorcinol.[15]

COLA

The cola (kola) nut of Africa has been used as a stimulant and ap-petizer since prehistoric times—just as chocolate has served the same purpose in tropical America. It is striking that the two foods are not only closely related botanically and allergenically but that both con-tain caffeine.

Cola became important in the Western world when John S. Pember-ton, an Atlanta, Georgia, druggist, concocted a preparation whose chief ingredients were cola nut extract and coca leaf extract. In 1891 Asa G. Chandler, also an Atlanta druggist, bought the rights to the mixture and was soon using it as the base of a soft drink. It was destined to become the fabulously successful Coca-Cola. Coca-Cola originally contained a trace of cocaine, but it has long since been removed from the small amount of cola leaf that is still used. Although the cola ex-tract that Coca-Cola (and other cola drinks) contains is minute, it is present in sufficient quantity to cause symptoms.

The following note in the British journal *Lancet* for October 4, 1890, suggests that the British may have "missed the boat" on the bonanza of cola drinks:

> Kola champagne is delicate in flavour and full in body and contains in each bottle, according to our analysis, not less than two grains of caf-feine, the active principle of tea and coffee. One bottle is, therefore, equal in stimulating and recuperative power to a breakfast cupful of

strong tea. The dietetic value of the kola nut was, we believe, first brought before the English public by Mr. Thomas Christy, and it is now well known that it is not only a valuable food, but also a nerve stimulant comparable only with tea. It appears to occupy a position between cocoa and tea, containing the nutritive ingredients of the former with the caffeine of the latter.[5]

COLLARDS

This non-heading variety of cabbage is widely grown in the Southern United States. Collards are closely related to kale, and the two are sometimes classed together as coleworts.[115]

COLORS, FOOD

As someone has put it, "Americans will eat anything if you manage to color it orange." He might have broadened his comment by saying we want color to match flavor. It would be impossible to market margarine if it were white and difficult to sell butter and most cheeses if they were of a pale ivory color. And no one would buy a grape drink if it was not colored purple, a cherry drink if it was not colored red, or an orange drink if it was not colored orange. According to a story coming out of World War II, a pilot from Florida had a large orange painted on the fuselage of his plane. That night, if we are to believe the story, a California pilot went out and painted "color added" across the orange.

Food colors may be either natural or synthetic. Both types are, of course, chemicals; so, indeed, are all substances. But the newer synthetic colors, not having the long record of proven safety, are under close scrutiny by governments everywhere. The main reason for such scrutiny is the possibility that they may be carcinogenic.

In ordinary home cookery, colors automatically and appropriately match the foods with which they are associated. Thus peas, spinach, and beans are naturally green; cherries and beets are naturally red; turnips and Irish potatoes are naturally white; and carrots, oranges, and sweet potatoes are naturally yellow or orange. But in commercial foods, since natural colors may be destroyed either in preparation or from sitting on the shelf, colors must be used to win consumer acceptance.

COLORS, NATURAL

Many foods are by nature strongly colored, and this adds much to their appeal. Examples are red apple, golden apple, peach, apricot, asparagus, beet, blueberry, broccoli, carrot, cherry, cheese, coffee, sweet corn, cranberry, egg, grape, lemon, lettuce, lime, butter, peppermint, mustard, orange, parsley, pea, peppers, pumpkin, radish, rhubarb, saffron, spinach, strawberry, sweet potato, and tomato. When a food is lacking in color, other plant (and, in the case of chochineal, animal) products may be borrowed to add the desired color. Since none of the synthetic colors in present use are oil-soluble, such products as butter, oils, cheese, salad dressings and margarines are colored either with carotenoids (beta-carotene and beta-apocarotenal) or annatto. Cochineal, a scarlet colorant derived from an insect, has been largely replaced by synthetic dyes. Another colorant classed as "natural" is caramel, which imparts a brown color to root beer, cola drinks, and rye bread.

Other natural colors are beet juice, fruit juice, grape skin extract, paprika, saffron, and turmeric. Of all natural colors the only one I have seen act as an allergen is turmeric.

COLORS, SYNTHETIC

Several synthetic dyes are used in such products as candies, icings, carbonated and still beverages, snack foods, pharmaceuticals, gelatin desserts, Popsickles, and baked goods. They are used in concentrations of 0.005% to 0.13%. Those certified by the Food and Drug Administration are listed in Table 5-3. The only dyes in widespread use, making up over 90% of the industrial output, are allura red (FD&C red #40), tartrazine (FD&C #5), and sunset yellow (FD&C #6). Their structural formulas are shown in Figure 5-1. FD&C *lakes* are insoluble colorants prepared by adsorbing dyes on aluminum hydroxide. They are probably not allergenic.

Table 5-3
FD&C Food Dyes

Permanent Listing	Provisional Listing
Tartrazine, FD&C Yellow #5	FD&C Red #4 (for coloring
Allura, FD&C Red #40	maraschino cherries)
(and lake)	FD&C Yellow #6
FD&C Blue #1	FD&C Blue #2
Orange B (for coloring	FD&C Green #3
sausage casings)	Lakes of FD&C colors
Citrus Red #2 (for color-	(except FD&C Red #40)
ing orange skins)	
Erythrosine, FD&C Red #3	

The question as to which dyes should be certified as safe is in a state of confusion, and no two countries have the same criteria. The cause of this confusion is the prevalent fear of many people that they are somehow being poisoned by food additives. This fear has been brought on (and kept alive) by popular books on additives, television talk-show "experts," radical consumer groups, and unwise legislation. For example, in 1976, the FDA, basing its action on extremely dubious studies and under public pressure, banned amaranth (former FD&C red #2). Amaranth has been replaced by allura red (FD&C #40), while in Canada amaranth is allowed and allura red is banned. A neutral observer, Darby, has commented, "Such divergent regularity actions from nation to nation reflect less the scientific evidence and its interpretation than the political and populace pressures brought to bear upon decision makers."[38]

The first case of sensitivity to a food dye seems to have been that reported by Baer.[11] His patient had a reaction resembling erythema multiforme caused by a green "aniline" dye. In 1958, I reported six cases of asthma caused by azo dyes.[174] In a later study of 39 cases, 24 reacted to red colors, 9 to yellow-orange, and 6 to both.[177] At that time the common red dye was amaranth (FD&C red #2), and the common dyes used to impart a yellow/orange color were tartrazine (FD&C yellow #5) and sunset yellow (FD&C yellow #6).

In 1959, Lockey reported three cases of allergy to tartrazine.[123] For some reason, sensitivity to dyes other than tartrazine has been neglected. Castelain has found the three most common offenders in France to rank as follows: erythrocine (a red dye used but little in the United States), 31 cases; "colors of plant origin," 28 cases; and tartrazine, 8 cases.[27] In the most recent study of aspirin allergy made by our group, only four (2%) of 205 aspirin-sensitive patients gave a history of reacting to yellow colors, while 7 (3.4%) reacted to red colors.[183] We agree that tartrazine is important and feel that it may be the most potent dye allergen. But it is not the most common.

Interest in tartrazine has led to the theory that it cross-reacts with aspirin. One study supports this: Juhlin et al reported that it caused adverse reactions in 7 of 8 aspirin-sensitive patients.[103] Their findings are not supported by the studies of others. Delaney found that only 3 of 40 aspirin-sensitive patients reacted to tartrazine.[42] Settipane and Pudupakkam found 6 cases in a series of 50,[165] Vedanthan et al found none in 5 cases,[205] and Weber et al found none in 45.[206] As stated above, our group found a history of reactions to yellow dyes in only 4 cases among 205 aspirin-sensitive patients.

Some observers carry further the theory that tartrazine cross-reacts with aspirin and believe that it is involved in the so-called triad of 1) aspirin sensitivity, 2) asthma, and 3) nasal polyps. This combination is said to signal a poor prognosis. This has not been the experience of our group, and we reject the concept of such a triad. As Weber at al say, "We feel that nasal polyps . . . and ASA intolerance are each associated with severe asthma and therefore are epiphenomena not necessarily related to each other. 'Triad asthma' is an attractive but misleading term."[206]

Consumers are confused as to the dyes they may encounter. Because of special attention being paid to tartrazine, manufacturers are required to list it on labels. Until this rule is applied to other dyes, patients must often guess. Some help may be obtained by checking common dye combinations as listed in Table 5-4.

Table 5-4
Color Combinations in Carbonated Beverages

Flavor	Color	Parts
Orange	FD&C Yellow #6	100
	or	
	FD&C Yellow #6	96
	FD&C Red #40	4
Cherry	FD&C Red #40	99.5
	FD&C Blue #1	0.5
Grape	FD&C Red #40	80
	FD&C Blue #1	20
Strawberry	FD&C Red #40	100
Lime	FD&C Yellow #5	95
	FD&C Blue #1	5
Lemon	FD&C Yellow #5	100

CORIANDER

Coriander is said to have a flavor somewhat reminiscent of lemon peel and sage. It is an important spice in sausages, including frankfurters, and is also used in curries. It is mentioned in Sanskrit writings of 1500 B.C. and in the Old Testament.

CORN (MAIZE)

This native American plant is the source of a grain that ranks near the top as a potent allergen. It is an especially common cause of headache, the tension-fatigue syndrome, and respiratory allergy. Unfortunately for those allergic to it, corn is more widely used than any other American food product. In fact, most prepared foods in our stores contain corn in one form or another. It appears as whole corn (corn on the cob and canned corn), cereals, hominy and grits, popcorn, Mexican foods (tacos, Fritos, enchiladas, tortillas), and as corn oil, meal, flour, starch, and syrup. It is used in the manufacture of beer, vinegar, and such whiskies as bourbon, Canadian, and of course, corn whisky.

Although a member of the grass family, corn does not cross-react with the related wheat, rice, rye, oats, and barley. However, patients with rhinitis from grasses will have trouble if they go into a corn field at the pollinating (tasseling) stage. Since corn pollen is the largest of all air-borne pollens, it does not affect patients except on such close contact.

Corn syrup is an especially important and potent corn allergen. A type of corn syrup containing a high proportion of fructose is coming into increasing use, especially in carbonated drinks. Its popularity with manufacturers is based on the fact that it is sweeter than other sugars and less expensive.

The fact that corn-sensitive patients react to corn syrup indicates that it is the presence of higher oligosaccharides that is responsible. These are known to be present in corn syrup. The fact that crystalline dextrose, used for intravenous administration, does not cause symptoms gives support to this assumption.

Corn oil is an occasional cause of symptoms in corn-sensitive patients. The widely held opinion that lipids are nonallergenic has obscured the importance of this corn product.

COTTONSEED

Cottonseed *oil* competes with soy oil and coconut oil for the American market. Cottonseed *flour* has been used to some extent to give fine texture to candies, pastries, and doughnuts. Cottonseed allergy, although rare, may be the most severe of all sensitivities; I have seen two such patients. In one case concerning a two-year-old boy, a scratch test resulted in anaphylactic shock. For this reason I no longer test for cottonseed, relying instead on the patient's history.

CRANBERRY

Although traditionally limited to the Thanksgiving holiday and other occasions when turkey is served, cranberry sauce is becoming a popular year-round food. Also increasing in use is cranberry juice, straight or mixed with apple juice. Allergy to cranberry is rare, so it makes a useful fruit for patients allergic to other fruits. Cranberry has many relatives, such as lingonberry, blueberry, and cowberry.

CRUSTACEANS

Perhaps because of its wide popularity, shrimp is the chief allergen in this group. However, there is no reason to believe that lobster, crayfish, and crab are not equally allergenic. Crustacean allergy is almost always severe, and patients can be expected to react to minute amounts. Its victims need no help in recognizing their problem or advice in avoiding exposure; only when they are accidentally exposed do they need the physician's assistance.

Shrimp and crab are often hidden in potato chip dips and in fancy fish dinners such as those served on the Gulf Coast.

Many crustacean-sensitive patients believe they are allergic to all seafood. But if they are allergic to oysters and other mollusks, abalone, or true vertebrate fish, the connection is purely a matter of chance. (See also Shrimp.)

CUCUMBER

Like other raw melons, raw cucumbers tend to cause gastric distress. Horticulturists, recognizing this tendency, have developed a "burpless" cucumber. Cucumber pickles do not seem to cause this problem.

CUMIN

This pungent spice (also known by its Spanish name *comino*) has been used since ancient times in all parts of the world. Isaiah (28:25) speaks of the plowman planting "cummin," and in Matthew 23:23 we read, . . . ye tithe of mint and anise and cumin. It it familiar to Americans because of the unique flavor it gives to Mexican food. It is also widely used by the peoples of the Mediterranean area and the Middle East. It is a fairly common allergen.

CURRANT

The term currant was originally applied to small raisins imported from the port of Corinth, hence the name. In the United States it usually refers to a red berry from various species of bushes closely related to gooseberry. Currants make delicious jelly. For some reason, they are now grown much less than formerly.

CURRY

Curries are highly spiced sauces used in the preparation of meats, fish, shrimp, chicken, and other foods, including rice. There is no standard curry powder, but most are said to contain various combinations of the following: allspice, turmeric, fenugreek, ginger, coriander, black pepper, cumin, nutmeg, clove, cinnamon, cardamom, and chili peppers.

DANDELION

When we think of the dandelion, we think of it as the most persistent and pernicious of all lawn weeds. But in many parts of the country, it is gathered for use as greens, and seed is available for growing it in the vegetable garden.

DASHEEN

The tubers of this relative of taro are used for food in the South Pacific.

DATE

Another food whose origin is lost in antiquity is the date, a delectable and nourishing fruit. Perhaps most Americans associate dates with figs, but the two fruits are not related. The date grows on a palm tree; the fig on a broad-leafed tree related to the mulberry and to the Osage orange, the "hedge apple tree" of the Midwest. Patients allergic to dates are usually, if not always, allergic to the coconut, also the fruit of a palm.

DAY LILY

Growing along country roads and in yards of abandoned farmhouses is the beautiful day lily, a flower with yellow-orange petals. This lily was introduced as a garden flower but has long since escaped from cultivation. It is one of the few plants whose flowers are used as foods.

Before the flowers open fully, they may be prepared for the table in the same way as are green beans. They also may be dried to be used later in soups. Their use in China in this way is widespread. The tubers, although small and tedious to prepare for cooking, are also edible.[29]

DILL

The only common use of dill (dillweed) is in the preparation of pickles made from such fruits as cucumber, tomato, and okra. Dill is one common member of the parsley family that I have not been able to identify as an allergen.

EGG

The hen's egg (and that of other poultry) is an excellent food. It is nourishing, delicious, and a valuable source of protein, vitamins, and iron. It has many uses in cookery. Unfortunately, however, it is also a common allergen capable of causing any of the reactions known to be caused by food allergy. It is often said that egg allergy is always severe. It is true that few allergens are capable of being as potent, but most patients have considerable tolerance, even being able to eat one egg every week or so.

One of the great dangers of egg allergy is that its victims, no matter how slight their degree of sensitivity, tend to have violent reactions to certain vaccines grown on chicken embryos. Some of these vaccines seem to be entirely free of egg protein contamination, but others, notably influenza vaccine, are not to be trusted.[39] As far as I can determine, all my egg-sensitive patients who have been given this vaccine have had adverse reactions, their chief symptoms being fever, prostration, and malaise. A recent egg-sensitive patient, a vigorous, stable young man, reported missing two weeks from work because of such a reaction.

EGGPLANT

Throughout the world, eggplant is one of the most widely used vegetables. It has never been especially popular in the United States, and for this reason I have had little experience with it as an allergen. However, I suspect that it cross-reacts closely with another fruit of the nightshade family, tomato. It is also known as eggapple, aubergine, and garden egg.

104

ELDERBERRY

This roadside weed produces an abundance of fruit, which may be used in making jelly and wine. The shoots, leaves, bark, and roots are poisonous.

EMULSIFIERS

Emulsifiers are used to disperse one liquid in another. Those that are now most commonly used in food manufacture are various monoglycerides and diglycerides. These agents emulsify oil in water and are used in maintaining the integrity of ice cream, margarines, shortenings, and baked goods. Sorbitan monostearate serves the same purpose. Various polysorbates are used to emulsify oil in water, thereby allowing essential oils to stay in suspension in soft drinks, ices, and sherbets. They also enhance the freezing qualities of ice cream. For over two centuries egg lecithin has been the emulsifier for mayonnaise. Soy lecithin is now used in many foods.

ENDIVE

Although our experience in this country with endive is limited, it seems to cross-react with lettuce, a related member of the sunflower family.

FENNEL

The leaves of this plant are used as a potherb, and its fruits ("seeds") are used in candy. It imparts a flavor similar to its relative anise. *Finnochio*, a Florentine variety, furnishes leaf stalks which, when blanched, have a flavor and consistency similar to the related celery.

FENUGREEK

The seed of this plant is ground and used as one of the strong spices of curry sauce. The leaves are also used in cooking, especially in the Orient.

FIDDLEHEAD FERN

The soft budding stems of fiddlehead fern, or cinnamon fern, are cooked like broccoli.

FIG

Although an important staple in the diet of many peoples of the world, the fig has never reached a high level of acceptance in this country. I have not seen a patient allergic to figs, and I often recommend it to patients who have multiple food allergy. I have no reference to fig allergy, but well over a century ago Nunn wrote, "A gentleman. . . informed me he could not eat figs without experiencing formication of the palate and fauces."[141]

FILBERT

Because it supposedly ripens on St. Philbert's day, August 22, the English named this nut the filbert. In the United States it is almost always known as the hazelnut. Some authorities apply the term filbert to the two species of European filbert, *Corylis cornuta* and *C. avellana* and reserve the term hazelnut for the American species, *C. americana*. I well remember one case of severe generalized urticaria brought on by a boy eating an ice cream supposedly containing almonds but which actually contained hazelnuts.

FINES HERBES

These are a mixture of parsley and chervil, finely chopped. Chives are sometimes included. They are used in omelettes and salads.

FISH

A fish may be defined as a vertebrate animal that possesses gills throughout life, which lives in the water, and whose limbs are modified as fins. This classification is close enough for our purposes. It clearly rules out aquatic mammals, amphibians, crustaceans, and mollusks. Fish allergy is fairly common and is almost always severe. No allergist need tell a patient he is allergic to fish; he already knows it. The only exception to this is the case of an infant with a strong skin reaction who has never tasted fish.

Tuft and Blumstein reported three patients whose allergy to fish was so severe that fish could not be brought into the house, nor could the patient visit a fish market.[197] Every allergist sees such patients. Erasmus, who wavered between Catholicism and the Reformation, was allergic to fish. He is said to have remarked, "My heart is Catholic, but my stomach is Lutheran."

By consulting the biological relationships of fish (Chapter 4), the patient allergic to one or more species may be able to see what species are sufficiently far removed biologically to be worth trying. This procedure is not, however, dependable. I have seen two patients who could eat red salmon but not pink salmon. Although in the same family, red salmon and pink salmon are different species. Most patients allergic to fish simply leave all fish alone, unless, of course, they know of kinds they are sure cause no trouble.

As Trager has pointed out, one of the confusing things to patients selecting fish is the wide number of common names often given to the same species. He writes:

> King mackerel may be sold as cero, silver cero, black salmon, cavalla or kingfish; but kingfish may also mean king whiting, which is sold as well under the names ground mullet, whiting, gulf whiting, surf whiting, southern whiting, sand whiting, and silver whiting. Just plain whiting, though, may be called silver hake.[195]

It would be impossible to list all edible fish, but I believe Table 5-5 is reasonably complete.

FLAVORS

Whether it is a food or not, every substance has some sort of flavor, but only a few are pleasant to the taste, and to the "picky eater," the list of these is short. Even the person who insists that he likes all foods will confess, if the point is pressed, that he likes some foods much more than others. Pressed further, he will probably admit that there are some flavors he does not like at all.

Because flavor is so important, the peoples of the world have always done all they can to make foods taste good, resorting to spices, sweeteners, salt, vinegar, and other additives. In recent years synthetic flavors are being used much more freely. There are several reasons for this, among which are economy and availability. It is said that all the natural vanilla in the world would be insufficient to flavor the vanilla ice cream eaten in the United States alone. And all the Concord grapes grown in this country could not possibly supply the flavor of the many artificial drinks, Popsicles, bubble gums, and other products that are supposed to taste like grapes.

Here is a list of some of the common artificial flavors; the flavors they provide or help provide are in parentheses: allyl caproate (pineapple), allyl disulfide (onion, garlic), anisic alcohol (peach), ben-

Table 5-5
Common Edible Fish

alewife	flounder	pompano
anchovy	grayling	porgy
barracuda	grouper	puffer
bass,	grunt	red snapper
many types	gudgeon	redfish
blackfish	haddock	roach
bluefish	hake	rockfish
bluegill	halibut	sailfish
bonito	herring,	salmon,
bullhead	many types	many types
butterfish	kingfish	sole
carp	mackerel	sprat
catfish,	menhaden	sturgeon
many types	mullet	sunfish
chub	muscolonge	swordfish
cod	perch	tarpon
crappie	sardine	trout
croaker	shad	tuna
dab	skate	turbot
dace	smelt	weakfish
dolphin	pickerel	whitefish
drum	pike	whiting
eel	pollack	

zaldehyde (cherry), ethyl acetate (strawberry), ethyl phenylacetate (honey), ethyl vanillin (vanilla), methyl anthranilate (orange), methyl salicylate (wintergreen), and phenylethyl acetate (rose).

The sound of these chemical names is frightening until we note the equally formidable list of chemicals that are naturally present in foods, chemicals that nobody worries about (this time the source of flavor is in parentheses): terpineiol (cardamom), sedenene (celery seed), cinnamic aldehyde (cinnamon), eugenol (clove), allyl isothiocyanate (horseradish and mustard), piperidine (black pepper), and thymol (thyme). No mother watching her child put mustard on his hot dog worries because it naturally contains allyl isothiocyanate. This does not mean that our government is not keeping a close eye on all food products. All food products are chemicals, whether they are produced by plants and animals or in the laboratory. Their wholesomeness is important to everyone.

FLAXSEED

Except for "Roman meal," which is used in breakfast cereals and bread, flaxseed (linseed) is a food that most people are not exposed to. I have not encountered a case of allergy to flaxseed, but that it can be the cause of violent allergic manifestations is revealed by these somewhat abridged letters, which were published in the *British Medical Journal* over a century ago:

> Dr. T. E. Clark writes: Some time ago (in 1858) I had under my care an old lady, aged 83, who not only suffered as if under the influence of asthma when the linseed-meal was applied to her person but would even say "that there was linseed-meal in the house, and that she knew it by the irritation in her nose and chest."[31]

> Dr. Diver writes: I recommended a man who consulted me a year or two ago to use a linseed-meal poultice, and he told me he dared not use it; nor, indeed, could he sit in his room if any linseed-meal were in the cupboard, for he got an attack of asthma under such circumstances.

> Another correspondent says: I have two nephews for whom linseed-meal poultices are never prescribed. Their application is invariably attended with irritation and oedema of the face. One of them, on sleeping in the same bed with a schoolfellow who had on a linseed-meal poultice, was affected in a like manner. I have not had any experience with regard to spasmodic asthma.[52]

In 1930 an article appeared which, as far as I can determine, contains the only reported cases of allergy to flaxseed in foods.[18] Two cases are reported. In one, the patient on eating Roman meal for the first time suddenly developed edema of the tongue and throat. This was followed by vomiting, hoarseness, nasal discharge, and conjunctival edema. The second case was marked by dyspnea, wheezing, urticaria, and cyanosis. This patient had had previous trouble from a flaxseed poultice.

GARBANZO

Although this legume has long been known as the chick pea or pulse, it is now generally given the Spanish name *garbanzo*. It probably cross-reacts completely with other mature seeds of the legume family. Golbert et al. reported the case of a man who was seen because of dizziness, dyspnea, wheezing, generalized pruritis, and facial and pharyngeal edema.[75] These symptoms came on while he was eating. The allergen proved to be partially cooked garbanzos. He apparently later had no trouble from them when they were properly cooked.

GARLIC

The bulblets (cloves) of this relative of onion are used throughout the world as a potent seasoning. It was part of the ration of the common Roman soldiers. This led some wag to remark that Roman troops may have been so successful partly because they knocked the enemy down with their breath. The chief allergic reaction to garlic is migraine, which is often severe.

GELATIN

Gelatin is a complex mixture of proteins used in desserts and candies and as a thickener and stabilizer. It is derived from the boiling of connective tissue, bones, and skin of beef and pork. I have not been able to see that it acts as an allergen.

GENIPAP

This is a tropical fruit grown in the West Indies and tropical South America. It may be eaten raw, but is more widely used as a conserve. A related fruit is the seven-year apple of Florida.

GINGER

The rhizomes of the ginger plant are the source of a spice used in such foods as baked goods (gingerbread and gingersnaps) and in ginger ale. However, patients who react to gingerbread usually react to the cinnamon it contains, not ginger. The whole rhizomes (ginger roots) are used extensively in Chinese dishes.

GOOSEBERRY

These tart berries are used in pies and jelly. They are closely related to currants.

GRANADILLA

The purple granadilla and the giant granadilla, tropical fruits of the passionflower family, are also known as passion fruits. Their sour-sweet taste is said to add much to the flavor of salads.

GRAPE

The several grape species and their hybrids are allergenically identical. They are eaten fresh and are also the source of grape juice, wine, vinegar, jellies, jams, and raisins. Although allergy to grape is unusual, it is characteristically severe.[24] One of my patients, a woman in her early forties, developed a constitutional reaction to a scratch test.

GRAPEFRUIT

Although closely related to orange, lemon, and other citrus fruits, grapefruit does not always cross-react with them.

GROUND CHERRIES

These are fruits of the nightshade family, closely related to tomatoes. Depending on the species, the fruits are yellowish or reddish; they are surrounded by a papery calyx resembling a lantern. Many are common weeds.

GUAVA

There are several varieties of this tropical fruit. Guava juice is sometimes available in the United States; it is delicious.

GUMS

As used in foods, gums are soluble plant polysaccharides and their derivatives. They are of great value in the food industry as emulsifiers and stabilizers and in imparting viscosity to such liquid products as salad dressings.[115] In Table 5-6 are listed food gums in common use.

HACKBERRY

The hackberry (sugarberry) grows on a common tree closely related to the elm. Gathering hackberries is hardly worth the trouble; they are best left for the birds.

HAZELNUT

(See Filbert.)

"HEALTH FOODS"

Throughout the world there is tremendous interest in so-called "health," "natural," or "organic" foods. If this idea were to be carried to its logical conclusion, we would exist on nothing but raw and unprocessed foods, including meats, eggs, fish, milk, vegetables, grains, and fruits. And we would be wide open to all sorts of bacterial infections, parasitic infestations, and plant toxins, not to mention chronic and intractable indigestion. But, fortunately for us, our remote ancestors discovered the virtues of roasting, frying, smoking, broiling, baking, stewing, fermentation, leavening, freezing, salting, pickling, and other such "artificial" procedures. They improved the appeal of foods with a variety of spices and such non-nutrient coloring materials as turmeric, saffron, and cochineal.

With the arrival of the industrial revolution, there was also a revolution in food manufacturing. The quality and safety of foods were extensively endangered, at times by ignorance, at other times by greed. In spite of present-day governmental control of food manufacturing, there is widespread suspicion that we are somehow being poisoned by processed foods. This is reflected in the spate of books on this subject to be found on the shelves of every public library. The result is the present health food craze.

As was true in the early days of the industrial revolution, ignorance and greed have arisen; ignorance on the part of the uninformed public, and greed on the part of promoters. In spite of claims by health food advocates, there are no guarantees that foods promoted as "organically grown" actually are, that they are grown without

Table 5-6
Common Food Gums

Gum	Plant	Family
Agar	*Gelidium* spp	Seaweed
Algin	*Macrocystis pyrifera*	Seaweed
Carrageenin	*Chondras crispus, Gigartina stellata*	Seaweed
Carob	*Ceratonia siliqua*	Pea
Guar	*Camposia teragonolobus*	Pea
Gum arabic	*Acacia* spp	Mimosa
Karaya	*Sterculia urens*	Cola
Pectin	*Citrus* spp	Citrus
Pectin	*Pyrus malus* (apple)	Apple
Tamarind	*Tamarindus indica*	Senna
Tragacanth	*Astragalus* spp	Pea

pesticides, herbicides, and chemical fertilizers. On one occasion, health foods purchased in New York were found to contain pesticide residues significantly higher than those found in ordinary foods.[90] Bender, after surveying health foods in England, commented, "Since lemons are not grown in this country it is questionable whether organic lemons are worth twice the price. They are claimed to be organically grown and free from chemical aids, but it is very doubtful whether such claims could be substantiated in any imported food."[16]

In spite of the best efforts of physicians, dieticians, governmental food authorities, or anyone else looking dispassionately at health foods, the movement shows no signs of fading from the scene. But it is the duty of every physician to point out to inquiring patients that the claims made for these products are doubtful, that they are inordinately expensive, and that food money is better spent on standard foods. But the fight is an uphill fight. As Bender points out, " 'Natural foods' have considerable appeal at a time of personal rebellion against regimentation, mass production, and the common battles with an impersonal bureaucracy."

Not only are health foods promoted as being purer and more nutritious, they are even promoted as of therapeutic value. Any physician who will take the occasion to visit a health food store incognito and listen to advice handed out will be amazed to what extent its employees dispense medical advice. And, along with pamphlets to be found there, he will find their advice has a pseudoscientific ring that is bound to impress the uninitiated. Herbert has well said, "Thousands of people have been misled by deceptive 'nutrition information' from nutritionists whose credentials and anecdotal claims fall apart under close scrutiny. Among the code phrases often used to promote 'nutritional' remedies of unproven safety and efficacy are 'orthomolecular nutrition,' 'ecologic nutrition,' and 'nutritional,' 'metabolic,' 'holistic,' 'unconventional,' 'alternative,' 'unorthodox,' and 'nontoxic' therapy."

HONEY

In helping ourselves to the honey so painstakingly gathered and stored by the honeybee, as we have done since the Stone Age, we have made available an excellent food. But the bee has frequently had her revenge. Painful stings are always a possibility, and severe allergy to bee stings is common. This can be serious, even fatal. (Under certain conditions honey is toxic, as discussed in Chapter 2.)

Nectar, the raw material of honey, is made up chiefly of sucrose, but thanks to the action of the enzyme invertase secreted by the bee, honey consists chiefly of dextrose and levulose. These hexoses are nonallergic. Honey also contains about 2% protein.[136,211] It is apparently because of these proteins, specific for the flower from which the nectar is gathered, that honey may cause allergic reactions. Strem and Stoesser suggest that it is the pollen proteins that make up the protein fraction of honey.[187]

In 1909, shortly after the term allergy was coined, Smith reported a case of what he called buckwheat poisoning.[169] His patient reported all sorts of ways that buckwheat made him ill, including eating wheat flour ground in the same mill with the buckwheat and the eating of buckwheat honey.

In North America the chief source of commercial honey is the pea family, especially clovers of various kinds. Beekeepers in the Midwest tell me that sweet clover, a common weed, is especially important. Alfalfa, also a legume, has been a leading source, but is so susceptible to disease that, in the Midwest at least, it is not now commonly planted.

My experience with allergy to honey is limited to cases in which there is obvious cross-reactivity with legumes. I have several patients allergic to honey who also react to every food of the legume family, including pea, green bean, soybean, common (navy, pinto, etc) bean, lima bean, peanut, and licorice.

The sources of wholesome honey embrace a great number of flowering plants. Table 5-7 lists the most common.

Table 5-7
Plant Sources of Honey

acacia	cotton	leatherwood	sage (salvia)
alfalfa	dandelion	lemon	sourwood
algaroba	dogwood	lima bean	Spanish needles
apple	desert blossoms	logwood	spearmint
asters	eucalyptus	lotus	star thistle
avocado	fireweed	mesquite	sumac
basswood	gallberry	milkweed	thyme
bird's foot	goldenrod	orange	tulip tree
trefoil	guajillo	pine	tupelo
black locust	heartsease	privet	white
blueberry	heather	rape	(sweet) clover
buckwheat	horsemint	raspberry	white gum
coffee	lavender	rosemary	wild rose

HOPS

The dried female flowers of the hop plant are used in brewing. They contribute flavor and aroma and are said to act as a preservative.[115] Since virtually any ingestant can act as an allergen, sensitivity to hops is a possibility. The usual cause of allergy to beer, however, appears to be either yeast, corn, or malt.

HOREHOUND

This member of the mint family is found in cough drops and old-fashioned horehound candy.

HORSERADISH

Although related to the radish, horseradish is a different plant. Used with discretion it adds a welcome piquancy to meats. Commercial horseradish is a mixture of horseradish, vinegar, cream, sugar, salt, and various seasonings.

HUCKLEBERRY

A wild variety of blueberry.

INSECTS

> Yet these may ye eat of every flying creeping thing that goeth on all four, which have legs above their feet to leap withal upon the earth. Even these of them ye may eat: the locust after his kind, the bald locust after his kind, and the grasshopper after his kind. Leviticus 11:21,22.

> And the same John had his raiment of camel's hair, and a leathern girdle about his loins; and his meat was locusts and wild honey. Matthew 3:4.

It is not only from Scripture that we know insects have long been used as foods. They are important sources of protein in the Mideast, Africa, Australia, Japan, Thailand, and Mexico. Among the species used are locusts, grasshoppers, cicadas, crickets, termites, cockroaches, beetles, palm weevils, and caterpillars. The eggs of waterbugs are used in parts of Mexico to prepare cakes called *ahuatle*. (See also Cochineal.)

Except that ants and grasshoppers are novelty foods, Brues is correct in saying that "the consumption of insects by members of our western civilizations is at the present time entirely unintentional on their part."[25] While I was serving on Guadalcanal during World War II, several men brought me bread containing weevils. I had to point out to them that it was almost impossible for the bakers to keep weevils out of the flour. One of the men, after hearing my explanation said, "Well, anyway, as the baker says, 'It's fresh meat.'"

According to the *Farm Journal*, insects are receiving current attention as possible foods for the hungry peoples of the world. If this proves feasible, we may expect allergic reactions. We already know insects may cause severe reactions by their bites and stings. Insect fragments, especially those of the caddis and may flies, may act as inhalant allergens. And insects are arthropods of the same phylum as the highly allergenic crustacea.

JACKFRUIT

This large (up to 50 pounds) Malay fruit is eaten raw, boiled, or fried. Its seeds are roasted like chestnuts.

JAVA PLUM

The Java plum, also known as jambolan, is one of the many tropical fruits of the myrtle family.

JERUSALEM ARTICHOKE

The tubers of this sunflower (which is only distantly related to the true artichoke) are cultivated in truck and home gardens and also are found in the wild state. They have a pleasant flavor but also an unfortunate tendency to cause flatulence, even to a greater extent than that caused by beans.

JUJUBE

The varieties of jujube, a fruit, are said to be popular in India, Malaysia, and China. An oil is extracted from the seeds.

JUNEBERRY

This fruit, also known as serviceberry, comes from a wild plant of our western states. It is used in tarts, pies, and jellies.

KIWI FRUIT

This fruit, originally known as Chinese gooseberry, is now extensively grown in New Zealand, and these enterprising people have named it after their national bird, the kiwi. Fine has reported a case of sensitivity to kiwi fruit, but, strange to say, his patient reacted to it as an inhalant not as a food. She could not peel it but could eat it.[62]

KOHLRABI

The thickened stem of this strange-looking member of the cabbage group is the edible part of one of our most neglected vegetables. It can be eaten either raw or cooked, but unlike many vegetables, is much more delicious when eaten raw.

KUMQUAT

The kumquat is a small citrus fruit used in preserves and candies.

LAMB

Because it is a minor source of meat in most of the United States, American allergists have little experience with lamb as an allergen. I have never seen lamb allergy except as a temporary intolerance in infants on lamb-based formulas.

LAMB'S QUARTERS (GOOSEFOOT)

Although as a weed of vegetable gardens it is a tremendous nuisance, this plant provides excellent greens. When picked early in the spring, the leaves have a flavor surpassing spinach. It also may be used uncooked in salads.

LAVER

Laver is a seaweed whose fronds are prepared for the table by pickling or stewing.

LEEK

This relative of the onion is similar in flavor but milder and sweeter. The parts used for food are the leaf stalks and leaves.

LEMON

The unique flavor of lemon, both the pulp and rind, adds much to many foods, drinks, and pastries. It is especially welcome when tartness is desired. The lime is closely related and can, from the allergic point of view, be considered the same fruit.

LEMON GRASS

Citral, the active principle of this aromatic grass, adds flavor to foods of Southeast Asia. It is grown in herb gardens in the United States.

LEMON VERBENA

This aromatic herb has leaves with a lemon-like flavor. Its chief use is in salads.

LENTIL

The shape of this small legume seed is that of a biconvex lens, hence the name. It is used in stews and soups. It has an especially high content of protein. Since it is not a common food, I cannot say whether or not it cross-reacts with other legumes, but I assume it does.

LETTUCE

Since it is the largest of the plant families, the sunflower (composite) family would be expected to furnish a large number of foods. It does not, however, and the only really common food plant of this family is lettuce. Lettuce seems to cross-react, at least to some extent, with such composite foods as artichoke and sunflower seed and with the pollens of the ragweeds, false ragweeds, sages, and other air-pollinated composites.

LICORICE

This legume provides a food not from its seed or fruit but from its roots. Considerable cross-reactivity prevails between licorice and the other legumes.

In 1968 Koster reported a case of severe hypertension caused by the ingestion of excessive amounts of licorice.[114] The patient's blood pressure was 220 over 140. It was estimated that he had been eating some 100 grams of licorice everyday. Licorice contains the steroidlike glycyrrhatinic acid, which acts like adrenal corticosteroids.

LIME

(See Lemon.)

LITCHI

According to Larn, this fruit is capable of causing asthma, angioedema, and nasal congestion. The dried fruit, often called litchi nut, causes less severe symptoms.[116]

LOQUAT

This small fruit of the apple family is sometimes cooked and served with other fruits in salads.

LOTUS

Both seeds and rhizomes of *Nelumbo nucifera,* the lotus of China, are used as food.

LOVAGE

The leaf, seed, and root of this herb are used as a flavoring agent.

MACADAMIA NUT

This native of Queensland, Australia, is both delicious and expensive. I know of no case in which it has acted as an allergen. This makes it useful to patients sensitive to other nuts.

MACE

(See Nutmeg.)

MALT

(See Beer.)

MANGO

This delicious peachlike fruit has been called the king of the tropical fruits. It is served raw in much the same way as cantaloupe and honeydew melon. It is also used in curries and jellies. As a member of the same family as poison ivy, oak, and sumac, mango may cause an equally severe contact dermatitis.

Ruben et al. have reported a case of anaphylactic shock caused by the ingestion of mango.[159] The patient developed chills, wheezing, difficulty in swallowing, and coma.

MANNA

The flowering manna tree of the Sinai desert produces a gum when its bark is injured. It soon dries and forms flakes. We read in Exodus 16:14,15:

> And when the dew that lay was gone up, behold, upon the face of the wilderness there lay a small round thing, as small as the hoar frost on the ground. And when the children of Israel saw it, they wist not what it was. And Moses said unto them, This is the bread which the Lord hath given you to eat.

(In Hebrew *man hu* means "what is it?")

MAPLE

Both maple and birch trees contain a sap rich in sugar. Maple sugar and syrup are valued for their distinctive flavor.

MARGARINES

The original oleomargarines were manufactured only as butter substitutes and marketed in similar packages. Now also available are soft margarines for spreading and liquid margarines for use on waffles, baked potatoes, and other foods. Margarines are made from the oils of soybean, cottonseed, corn, safflower, and peanut. By law, margarines are required to contain at least 15,000 International Units of vitamin A per pound.[129] Some brands add 2,000 International Units of vitamin D. Margarines are generally colored with beta carotene, not, as is often said, with the azo dye tartrazine.

MARJORAM

Marjoram is another of the many members of the mint family whose leaves are used as a spice. It is used in vegetable dishes, especially with lima beans, peas, and string beans. It is also said to add an agreeable flavor to lamb. It is found in some liverwurst and bologna.

MARSHMALLOW

Formerly used in the manufacture of candy, marshmallow, a relative of cotton and okra, is no longer used in the candies marketed as "marshmallows." Their base is gelatin and corn starch.

MATÉ (SPANISH, *YERBA MATE*)

Of the many plants that contain caffeine, one is this holly of Argentina and Paraguay. The leaves and shoots are used to make a caffeine-containing drink similar to tea.

MEAT SEASONINGS

There is probably no spice that may not be used (and has not been used) to season meats. In the case of the many kinds of sausage, black pepper and sage appear to be basic. Other spices that may be used are red pepper, anise, white pepper, Jamaica ginger, mace, thyme, mustard, coriander, onion powder, nutmeg, celery seed, cardamom, marjoram, and paprika.[219]

MEAT TENDERIZERS

These are proteolytic enzymes used to make inferior grades of meat more tender. The four in present use are papain, derived from papaya, ficin, derived from fig, bromelain, derived from pineapple, and fungal proteases.[219]

MILK

Although the word milk ordinarily means cow's milk, it applies, of course, to the milk of any mammal, including human milk. Goat's milk is used somewhat in the United States, and in various parts of the world milk is obtained from the ewe, buffalo, mare, yak, camel, and reindeer. A tremendous variety of cheese is derived from these milks.

In this discussion we are concerned with cow's milk, but goat's milk, if not allergenically identical,is so close that no separate discussion is necessary.

It is safe to say that people who use animal milks have known from the beginning that they are made up of curds and whey. We now know that they are a mixture of proteins, fats, lactose (sugar of milk), salts, vitamins, and water.

It is the proteins that concern us. According to Goldman et al, each 100 ml of milk contains the following proteins: casein, 2,800 mg; beta-lactoglobulin, 420 mg; alpha-lactalbumin, 70 mg; serum albumin (bovine serum albumin or BSA), 20 mg.[76]

Although milk proteins undoubtedly are the cause of true milk allergy, some infants show intolerance to butterfat, and it is possible (but difficult to prove) that trace chemicals introduced into milk by the animal's diet can cause trouble.

Cow's milk is the undisputed "king" of the food allergens. It is not only the most common in all age groups, but also causes an unusually large variety of symptoms. Since it ordinarily does not cause severe symptoms, at least in patients over one year of age, milk allergy is easily overlooked. The physician who watches constantly for milk allergy will find that it is amazingly common.

A rare but important phenomenon is severe allergy to traces of penicillin present in milk.[212] I have seen one such case; this patient also has had trouble from moldy bread and blue cheese.

MILLET

A large number of grasses furnish the millets, small seeds used in many parts of the world as food. In the United States their use is pretty much limited to organic food enthusiasts.

MINT

The plants most commonly known as mints are spearmint and peppermint, but the family includes such important spices as sage and thyme. All mints are aromatic and all have stems that are square in cross section.

MOLD INHIBITORS

Mold growth has always been a problem in baking. Among the most commonly used inhibitors are sodium diacetate, calcium propionate, and sodium propionate. In rare instances patients are so sensitive to penicillin that molds in bread may cause a reaction—I have recently seen such a case. Mold in bread can also cause trouble in patients allergic to such air-borne molds as *Alternaria*. But most important of all, if bakers did not use mold inhibitors, there would be widespread spoilage, with the result that bread prices would go even higher than they are now.

MOLLUSKS

Among the mollusks, the most commonly eaten are oyster, clam, abalone, snail, octopus, and squid. Also of some importance are scallop, mussel, cockle, and periwinkle. In the United States two bivalves, oyster and clam, are the most common mollusk allergens. They are inclined to cause severe reactions.

Uncommon mollusks are ormer, limpet, and piddock.

MONOSODIUM GLUTAMATE

As pointed out in Chapter 2, monosodium glutamate, a popular flavor enhancer, often causes "the Chinese restaurant syndrome." Two cases have been reported in which it caused severe asthma.[2]

MULBERRY

The red mulberry, a common weedy tree, produces the familiar mulberry. Although sometimes used in pies and jellies, mulberry is not a popular fruit.

MUSHROOM

The mushroom of commerce is *Agaricus bisporus*, closely related to the wild mushroom, *A. campestris*. Many other wild mushrooms are edible, but since it is difficult to differentiate them from poisonous types, gathering wild mushrooms is unwise. Hardin and Arena quote the old saying, "There are old mushroom hunters, and there are bold mushroom hunters. But there are no old, bold mushroom hunters."[83] I have recently seen several cases of allergy to morel (*Morschella esculenta*), a wild mushroom.

MUSTARD

Mustard is a member of a large family of food plants and weeds. Mustard seed is a spice used in prepared meats, sausages, chili, and the "prepared mustard" universally associated with the American hot dog. It is also used in the preparation of sardines. It is seldom allergenic.

NASTURTIUM

Young leaves of nasturtium are sometimes added to salads, and the buds of flowers are sometimes pickled and used in the place of capers.

NEW ZEALAND SPINACH

This plant is similar in appearance and flavor to true spinach but is a member of another family. It is much more easily grown than true spinach and has the advantage of thriving in hot weather.

NUTMEG AND MACE

Several trees of the genus *Myristica* produce a fruit whose seed is nutmeg and whose aril is mace. Nutmeg in high dosage is a dangerous hallucinogen.[78]

OATS

Dr. Johnson's definition of oats—a grain which is generally given to horses, but in Scotland supports the people—may have been true, but it is a popular ingredient of hot and cold cereals and cookies in the United States. Like any grain it may cause allergic reactions. It is not especially close to the other grains allergenically and occasionally is the only grain causing trouble.

OILS

Edible oils are derived from cottonseed, soybean, corn, rapeseed, coconut, palm kernel, palm husk, olive, sunflower seed, cocoa butter, peanut, and safflower. Although as lipids oils are theoretically nonallergenic, reactions are not uncommon and may be severe. The most important are cottonseed oil, peanut oil, and soy oil.

OKRA (GUMBO)

Few vegetables add more to a soup or stew than okra. (Botanically it is a fruit, but gastronomically it is used as a vegetable.) Its mucilaginous character, which is distasteful to many people, is useful in adding body to dishes made up of meat and mixed vegetables; its seeds add both nourishment and flavor.

ONION

The lowly onion has for ages added zest to a diet that might otherwise be flat and monotonous. Onions have, however, little food value. They are fairly common allergens, being especially important in causing headache and gastrointestinal distress.

ORANGE

The orange, including its varieties mandarin and tangerine, is rightfully popular. Unfortunately, all citrus fruits cross-react to a large extent, especially in eczema, so the orange-sensitive patient must usually avoid lemon, lime, grapefruit, and other citrus fruits.

Bendersky and Lupas report a case of anaphylaxis from orange.[17] The patient ate an orange at noon. At 2 PM he developed generalized itching, dizziness, excessive thirst, and chills. He then went into shock. He had a previous history of urticaria after eating an orange.

Patients often ask if citric acid is the troublemaker. This is rarely the case. When it is, the patient can usually identify its presence in pineapple and such products as carbonated drinks, candies, gelatin desserts, and other tart drinks and foods.

OREGANO

Also called wild marjoram, oregano is an essential ingredient of Mexican and Italian cookery, giving these foods their unique character. It is also popular with cooks of other nations.

OTAHEITE APPLE

This is a pear-shaped fruit grown extensively in Jamaica. It is also known as Malay apple.

PAPAYA

The tropical papaya tree grows readily in the wild but is also cultivated. The fruit, which resembles a melon or acorn squash, furnishes papain, an enzyme related to pepsin with similar proteolytic properties. It is therefore useful as a meat tenderizer. In some parts of the world it is known as papaw, a term reserved in the United States for a member of the custard apple family.

PAPAW

The custard apple family furnishes many fruits, but the only member to grow in North America is the pawpaw or pawpaw. It grows only in the wild; it is said to have a flavor similar to banana but less tempting.

PARSLEY

Parsley is used less as a seasoning than as a garnish, being more attractive than flavorful.

PARSNIP

This close relative of the carrot deserves to be used more than it is. Properly prepared, it can be delicious.

PASSION FRUIT

(See Granadilla.)

PEA

Unless it has a modifying adjective, the term pea refers to the seed of the common garden pea. It is a climbing leguminous plant, widely grown in home gardens and available in the market fresh, canned, or frozen. Many other legumes are known as peas, examples being crowder pea, black-eyed pea, pigeon pea, and cowpea. Most of these are more closely related to the common bean than to the pea.

The pea is less likely to cause allergic reactions than other legumes, but Edwards and Helming studied the case of a 24-year-old soldier who developed the following symptoms from eating soup containing peas: stertorous breathing, vomiting, cyanosis, involuntary urination, and coma.[57] He had had similar reactions previously from both pea and various types of beans. Even the odor of peas cooking would cause minor symptoms.

Allergy to peas is occasionally severe. It is, in fact, not uncommon for almost any seed allergens, such as cottonseed, peanut, buckwheat, and walnut, to cause severe reactions.

PEACH

If the peach is not the most delicious of all fruits, especially when eaten raw, it certainly is at the top of the list. Unfortunately, however, it is when eaten raw that it is most likely to act as an allergen.

PEANUT

As far as I have been able to determine, the peanut plant is unique in that it flowers above ground and forms its fruit below ground. It may be cooked in the same way as the common bean, but is commonly eaten roasted or in the form of peanut butter and peanut oil. Peanuts and peanut butter are used in candies (especially candy bars), cookies, and other baked goods.

Of all the legumes, peanut is the most likely to act as an allergen, and the reactions it causes are characteristically severe. As a result, the sensitivity is so obvious that the patient himself usually makes the etiologic diagnosis. Peanut can cause almost any type of allergic disorder, being commonly involved in asthma, headache, eczema, urticaria, and, occasionally, shock. It cross-reacts in many cases with other legumes, especially with its close relative soybean. (See also Oils.)

PECAN

This American relative of the hickory nut is a fairly common allergen. Although a member of the same family as the walnuts, there is little cross-reactivity. However, the patient allergic to one member of the walnut family should be suspicious of the others.

PEPPERS

The term pepper is confusing. It originally referred to a dried fruit now commonly known as black pepper. Explorers to the New World found Indians using fruits of the nightshades which had something of the flavor, piquancy, and tang of the pepper with which they were familiar. In 1493 Peter Martyr wrote that Columbus brought home with him "pepper more pungent than that from Caucasus."

Some peppers are sweet and mild, such as bell (mango) pepper and some of the banana peppers. Others, especially the cayenne and Tabasco peppers so popular in Mexico, are the familiar "hot peppers." Although related to tomatoes, potatoes, and eggplant, peppers cross-react with them very little, if at all. Many persons, however, find all types of peppers to be indigestible, even the sweet varieties.

PERSIMMON

When anyone who has gone into the woods to gather persimmons is asked about them, his first comment is likely to be that before they have ripened thoroughly, they are extremely puckery. Their flavor is somewhat similar to that of apricots and figs. One variety is kaki, the Japanese persimmon.

PINEAPPLE

Although pineapple has a flavor somewhat similar to that of the citrus fruits and is rich in citric acid, it belongs to another family and is the only food plant in that family. It is not an important allergen but often causes gastrointestinal distress, especially when eaten uncooked.

PINYON NUT

Several species of American pines produce this delicious nut. It is also known as piñon or pine nut. Other pine nuts are the monkey nut of Chile, parana of Brazil, and the bunya-bunya of Queensland.[115]

PISTACHIO

I have not seen allergy to this expensive but delicious nut, a relative of the cashew nut.

PLANTAIN

The term plantain is applied to a variety of banana used as a cooked vegetable. As far as I know its use is limited to the tropics. The term plantain is also applied to several species of unrelated lawn weeds.

PLUM

Plums are eaten either raw or cooked and in the dried state (prune).
I have no record of allergy to plum, prune, or prune juice.

POKE (POKEWEED)

The shoots of this wild plant are sometimes used as greens. The
roots are poisonous.

POMEGRANATE

When the spies of the Children of Israel returned to show Moses
and Aaron the richness of the Promised Land, they brought grapes,
figs, and pomegranates. And when in The Song of Solomon the lover
tries to find words to describe his beloved, he says, "A garden en-
closed is my sister, my spouse. . . . Thy plants are an orchard of
pomegranates with pleasant fruits." 4:12,13 Anyone who has tasted
pomegranates will agree that they are indeed delicious.

POPPYSEED

These seeds are used to add flavor and attractiveness to rolls and
breads. The opium poppy is not used for this purpose, but it could be
since its seeds do not contain opium.

PORK

Patients allergic to pork and ham almost always are already aware
of the fact before they seek medical advice, but they may overlook it
in prepared meats or in bits of sausage on pizza. Although both beef
and pork are mammalian meats, there is little cross-reactivity. One
can therefore usually be used as a substitute for the other. Some
patients tolerate cured meats like ham but cannot eat fresh pork,
especially pork roast.

POTATO

The Irish or white potato is related to the tomato, pepper, and
eggplant but not to the sweet potato. The potato is not a common
allergen, and when it is, the symptoms are usually mild. It can,
however, cause severe reactions; this is demonstrated by the following case reported just over a century ago:

The following curious case of idiosyncrasy came under my notice lately. Mrs. R., aged 35, widow, a person of somewhat spare habit and active disposition, informs me that, since childhood, she has had a very strong aversion for *potatoes*. She knows no reason for this aversion; certainly it is not due to any fanciful notion. It is the result, apparently, of a peculiar idiosyncrasy. When she was quite a little girl, her uncle was very fond of playing a trick on her by concealing a small morsel of potato in a bit of butter, and inducing her to take it. The result always was *very severe vomiting*. She remembers her mother being very angry with her uncle on the occasion when he indulged in this practical joke. If she happened to be present where potatoes were being cooked, she became quite faint; and, until within a few years back, she could not even handle the tubers. At present she would rather take the vilest medicines than taste a potato; indeed, she could not bring herself to do the latter.[1]

A common cause of "housewife's eczema" is peeling potatoes and slicing tomatoes. And the odor of potato has been reported as a cause of respiratory symptoms.[96]

PRESERVATIVES

Perhaps no food additives are more inclined to raise suspicion of harm than preservatives. At one time they were a real threat to health, and long after the Civil War, talk was still heard of the "embalmed beef" sent to the Union forces. As late as 1887 the *Journal of the American Medical Association* could report that the following agents were in use: Prussian blue, carbonate of copper, arsenite of copper, lead chromate, sulfuric acid, hydrochloric acid, and creosote.[56] Most of them probably were used to produce color, but they would certainly have retarded bacterial growth.[56]

The preservatives used in today's foods, so closely watched by government agencies, have all been carefully tested and cleared as safe. At times, however, there is doubt as to possible toxicity of some of them. A case in point is the use of nitrites in prepared meat and fish products. In the United States sodium or potassium nitrite may be added to meat at the rate of up to 3½ ounces per 100 pounds of meat. Nitrites occur naturally in spinach, beets, radishes, celery, and many other vegetables, and they appear often at significant levels in drinking water. Nitrites react with body amino acids to form nitrosamines, which are considered possible carcinogens. However, in a carefully documented review, Wolff and Wasserman point out that the possible carcinogenicity of nitrites is very much less than is the danger of botulism when nitrites are not used.[216]

Many patients ask about preservatives and other food additives. It is clearly the duty of physicians to point out to these people, especially when they have been frightened by extremists, that the Department of Agriculture and the Food and Drug Administration are cooperating with food producers to make our foods as safe and nutritious as possible.

PRICKLY PEAR

This fruit of the common cactus of arid areas of North America is sometimes used as a food. It is often seen in Mexican markets.

PUMPKIN

This melon is botanically a winter squash and resembles the other members of the species in both appearance and flavor. When a patient reports pumpkin allergy, it almost always turns out that the actual offender is cinnamon, which is used so freely in pumpkin pie. Allergy to pumpkin itself is rare. Roasted pumpkin seeds are a popular delicacy.

QUINCE

This member of the apple family, closely related to the pear, can properly be called an old-fashioned fruit. It was formerly used to prepare a type of jam known as quince honey.

RABBIT

Both the wild rabbit (cottontail) and the rabbit of the meat market are actually hares. I have not seen allergy to rabbit, but the following case report, published in 1883, shows that it has long been known to cause allergic reactions:

> I had the opportunity of witnessing the most interesting case of acute urticaria and spasmodic asthma I have ever seen the other evening whilst dining, showing how idiosyncrasy in certain articles of food affects certain individuals. A young lady was sitting at dinner, apparently in perfect health. She partook, amongst other things, of some rabbit, and in about ten minutes or so after she had eaten of it she was attacked with acute urticaria, showing large erythematous patches and wheals very prominent on face and neck. She then was seized with violent attacks of spasmodic asthma, which obliged her to leave the table. I inquired if she had ever suffered this before, and she informed me that she had after eating hare.[185]

RADISH

The many varieties of this root vegetable tend to cause indigestion in many people but seldom cause true allergic reactions. The Japanese field type, which is used as a cooked vegetable, is said to reach a weight as great as two pounds.

RAPE

The seed of this member of the mustard family is used in the Orient to produce salad oil.

RASPBERRY

Black and red raspberries are not berries but conglomerate fruits. Each seed, which so easily gets between our teeth, represents the seed of an individual fruit. Although related to the strawberry, the raspberry is not nearly so important in allergy. This may be because it is not as popular. (See also Blackberry.)

RHUBARB

The leaf stalks of this plant, although a vegetable, are used like a fruit in pies, sauces, and wine. The leaves themselves have long been considered to be toxic, but a review by Fassett does not support this.[59] Whether or not rhubarb and its relative buckwheat cross-react I cannot say from my experience, but the following report of Unger suggests that they do:

> A boy of 2 with severe asthma gave positive tests to only two antigens, buckwheat and rhubarb. The average person would not suspect that they are the two members of the *Polygonaceae* (buckwheat) family. The child was eating buckwheat cereal (kasha); rhubarb was added to his spinach to make it more palatable. Elimination of both brought prompt relief.[201]

RICE

Probably the most widespread misapprehension in the field of food allergy is that rice is hypoallergenic. In my experience it is almost as common an offender as its close relative wheat. In fact, the patient allergic to one is usually allergic to the other and also to barley. I ask patients who are allergic to wheat either to avoid barley and rice altogether or to be highly suspicious of them. The following cases were reported by Nunn in 1859:

> JM, an occasional patient, cannot eat rice in any shape without extreme distress. From the description given of his symptoms, I believe spasmodic asthma to be the cause of his discomfort. On one occasion, when at a dinner party, he felt the symptoms of rice-poisoning come on, and was, as usual, obliged to retire from the table, although he had not partaken of any dish ostensibly containing rice. It appeared, on investigation, that some white soup, with which he had commenced his dinner, had been thickened with ground rice.
>
> A gentleman who, as in the preceding case, could not eat rice "without being suffocated," took luncheon with a friend in chambers. The fare was simple—bread, cheese, and *bottled* beer. On the usual symptoms of rice-poisoning seizing him, he informed his friend of his peculiarity of constitution. The symptoms were explained by the circumstance of a few grains of rice having been put into each bottle of beer for the purpose of exciting a secondary fermentation.[141]

RUTABAGA

This root vegetable is related to the turnip, but its flavor more closely resembles that of the parsnip. It deserves to be used much more than it is. In Britain, rutabagas are known as swedes.

RYE

Rye is an occasional cause of severe reactions. It cross-reacts very little with its relatives in the grass family and for that reason is often useful as a substitute for wheat. Both American and Scandinavian rye crackers and crisp bread are available in many stores, and an acceptable rye bread can be baked at home. (See Chapter 8.) The rye bread sold in supermarkets, however, contains more wheat flour than rye flour.

Wherever rye is grown, a careful watch is made for ergot. Epidemics of poisoning by ergot of rye were reported in Russia in 1926, in Ireland in 1929, and in France in 1953.[22]

SACCHARIN

With the banning of the cyclamates, saccharin remains the only artificial sweetener. Saccharin itself has since been banned by the FDA. At this writing, however, final action is withheld pending further study by the Congress. I have not been able to demonstrate a definite case of allergy to this chemical.

SAFFLOWER

The oil of the seed of safflower, a member of the sunflower family, is now available. It can be used as a substitute oil by patients unable to take corn, cottonseed, soy, or peanut oil.

SAFFRON

This precious spice consists of the dried stigmas of a crocus now grown chiefly in Spain. It is valued both for its yellow color and pleasantly bitter flavor. It is a necessary ingredient of the Spanish dish *arroz con pollo* (rice with chicken).

SAGE

The term sage is applied to a number of weeds of the sunflower family, which, incidentally, are important sources of allergenic pollen. But the food plant known as sage is a mint, and it is a fairly common allergen. Patients often notice that it causes trouble when encountered in turkey dressing but are unaware that it is also found in prepared meats. It cross-reacts closely, if not perfectly, with other members of the mint family.

SAGO

The pith of the sago palm is the source of grains of starch used at times in soups. Some sago is obtained from cycads, plants intermediate between ferns and palms.

SALICYLATES

The chief sources of natural salicylic acid and its salts are the willows and their relatives, the *Salicaceae.* It has been said that other plants containing salicylates might cause trouble in patients allergic to aspirin (acetylsalicylic acid). South has exploded the possibility of removing salicylates from the diet by reporting that all except 3 of 60 different plants tested were found to contain them. She believes that all plants probably contain some salicylate and adds this wry comment: "Many foods now restricted by existing diet plans and which the patient wouldn't miss much (such as parsley, 1×10^{-2} mg/gm) contain roughly the same amount of salicylate as some presently restricted foods which are sorely missed by the patient (like strawberries, 4×10^{-4} mg/gm)."[172]

Further evidence that salicylates may be found naturally in all plants is supported by a study made by the Del Monte corporation.[192] Although minute traces were found in all 39 products studied, in no case was the level higher than a little less than one part per million. When we reflect on the fact that aspirin is the only salicylate known to cause allergic diseases and that no food contains more than scant amounts of salicylates, the folly of trying to prescribe foods free of salicylates is exposed.

SALSIFY

Salsify, also called oyster plant or goat's beard, is used as a root vegetable. It resembles parsnip in appearance but is supposed to resemble oyster in flavor. Whenever anyone sees a seed head rising from a weed patch that resembles the globular seed head of a dandelion (but is much larger), he is looking at a salsify plant. The seed head is the apparent source of the name goat's beard.

SAMPHIRE

This herb is used in parts of southern Europe for pickling, in salads, or as a potherb. The name is a corruption of the French *herbe de Sainte Pierre.*

SAPODILLA

This tropical tree supplies both a delicious fruit and the chewing gum base chicle. (See Chewing Gum.)

SARSAPARILLA

The root stocks of this plant are the source of a flavoring agent sometimes used in root beer.

SASSAFRAS

Another ingredient of root beer, sassafras, contains safrole, a chemical known to be carcinogenic. Other foods in which safrole is found are cinnamon, cocoa, mace, black pepper, and nutmeg. Fortunately, it appears in all these products in minute amounts, and they are therefore considered safe for use in foods and beverages. (Chemically pure safrole was formerly added to root beer at a level of 20 parts per million. This deliberate addition is no longer permitted.)

SAVORY

Savory is a flavoring agent of the mint family closely related to thyme.

SEQUESTRANTS

Sequestrants, also called chelating agents and metal scavengers, are used to deactivate or "sequester" metals such as copper and iron. These metals are undesirable in soft drinks because they tend to settle out and cloud them. They also tend to catalyze oxidation of foods, especially fats and oils.

The leading sequestrants are citric acid, sodium hexametaphosphate, and the salts of ethylenediaminetetraacetic acid (EDTA). The EDTA salts are used ·to sequester trace amounts of iron in beer, thereby preventing a sudden gush of foam when the can or bottle is opened. They react with several metals to inhibit off-taste, discoloration, or rancidity in canned shrimp, sandwich spreads, potato salads, mayonnaise, canned beans, and other items.

SESAME

To most of us, perhaps, our first thought when we hear the word sesame is either "Sesame Street" or the "open sesame" of *Ali Baba and the Forty Thieves*. But sesame is now in wide use as whole seed, ground seed, and oil. Torsney has reported three serious reactions.[194]

SHALLOT

Shallot is related to onion and garlic with a flavor resembling both.

SHRIMP

Shrimp has long been known to be a potent and common allergen. Nunn, writing in 1859, commented: "A personal friend of my own suffered from erythema nodosum after eating shrimps, although they were perfectly safe."[141] We would probably now call the patient's reaction urticaria.

My own case is an example of how serious shrimp allergy can be. I ate them for the first time at the age of 16. The immediate reaction was severe angioedema of the lips, mouth, and tongue. Once at a hospital staff dinner I ate a radish that was in the same dish with shrimp. I became so hoarse and developed so much lip edema that I was obliged to leave the meeting. On one occasion while playing two-handed pitch with my son, I began to notice severe itching and redness of my eyes. It turned out that my son had been eating shrimp with his fingers. The allergen had been transferred from his hands to the cards, thence to my hands, and finally to my eyes. Since then we do not bring shrimp into our house, nor do I have much enthusiasm for eating in seafood restaurants. Crustaceans closely related to shrimp are prawn, crayfish, scampi, and skirret.

SLOE

This relative of the cherry is used in flavoring sloe gin and, to some extent, as a preserve. It is also known as the blackthorn and is thought to be an ancestor of the plum.

SNAILS

Snails (*escargots* in France, *karicollen* in Belgium) are gourmet foods eaten in some European countries and to some extent in the United States.

SORGHUMS

There are many sorghums, but in the Midwest, at least, the term is ordinarily used for the sweet sorghums whose stems produce sorghum molasses. The other sorghums are an important source of food in many parts of the world, especially in Africa. Milo maise, commonly called simply milo, is one of the most widely grown small grain crops in the arid parts of the United States. In this country it is used chiefly in feeds for hogs and chickens but not in human food.

SOYBEAN

This legume, a comparative newcomer to North America, has become one of our most widely used foods and one of our most valuable agricultural products. Among some of its many uses are: green vegetable, infant formulas, flakes, grits, macaroni, spaghetti, bean sprouts (also obtained from mung beans), coffee substitutes, soy sauce, soy flour, bean curd, salad oil, cooking oil, margarines, shortenings, and lecithin. Soy isolates are now being used in making "meat extenders" and synthetic meatlike products. They are also commonly added to bread and other baked goods.

Because soybeans have long been used as the basis of formulas for infants unable to take cow's milk, they are often said to be hypoallergenic. Unfortunately, this is not true. The soybean is closely related biologically and allergenically to peanut and is nearly as allergenic.

The increasing use of two food products, soybean and corn syrup, is making the work of the allergist more and more difficult. It also makes life harder for patients unfortunate enough to be allergic to them. Few manufactured foods are free of one or the other, and many contain both.

SPINACH

Spinach is rarely allergenic. Although related to beet and Swiss chard, there is little evidence of cross-reactivity.

SQUASH

Summer and winter squash are among the least allergenic of vegetables and deserve to be used more commonly by highly allergic patients. They are easily grown in the home garden.

STABILIZERS AND THICKENERS

Those who remember peanut butter with oil floating on the top of the jar and chocolate milk with the chocolate settled on the bottom will appreciate the worth of these food additives. They serve a similar function in ice cream, cheese spreads, pie fillings, and syrups. As Trager has said, we now seldom see the warning "shake well before using" on food items.[195] The common additives of this class are gum arabic, gum guar, carob bean gum, carageenin, gelatin, gum tragacanth, and carboxymethylcellulose.

STAR ANISE

This spice is popular in China and Japan. It is botanically unrelated to true anise.

STAR APPLE

This fruit of a West Indian tree is said to be delicious when fully ripe but acrid and astringent when it is not.

STRAWBERRY

It is probable that most people will develop urticaria if they eat enough fresh strawberries. It is theorized that they are histamine releasers, but I know of no confirmatory evidence. Strawberry can also act as a true allergen; one of my patients insists that she has trouble from strawberries only when they have been cooked.

In 1917, before the term allergy had come into general use (or the concept was generally accepted), Schuyler reported this case:

> I recall one child seven or eight years of age who always had an aversion to strawberries; he claimed that they always made him sick. If he ate even one he always broke out with hives or something of that type. His parents believed that this refusal to eat strawberries was just a whim, and the father offered the boy a dollar if he would eat a certain number of strawberries. The boy managed to get three berries down, probably swallowing them whole. He became so sick that he almost died. He only recovered after a great deal of work on the part of the physician.[163]

Two years before, Frost reported a similar case of what we now call anaphylaxis to strawberry.[70] Five minutes after eating fresh strawberries a young woman developed generalized swelling and erythema, swelling of the tongue, and extreme respiratory embarrassment. Tracheotomy was considered, but the patient recovered after receiving 1 cc of epinephrine, 1-1,000. She had had a similar reaction from eating fresh strawberries one week before.

SUGARCANE

This grass is the source of most of the sugar consumed in the world. The pure white (granulated) sugar is not allergenic. Patients may have trouble, however, from brown sugar and from cane (and sorghum) molasses. Cane and sorghum are large grasses morphologically similar to corn, and cross reactivity among the three occurs.

SUGARS

Pure crystalline sugars, whether they are derived from cane, beet, or corn, do not act as allergens. An occasional patient complains of vague constitutional symptoms after consuming a significant amount of sugar. This should suggest the possibility of reactive hypoglycemia. It is fortunate that the corn-derived glucose (dextrose) so widely used parenterally is nonallergenic. Otherwise the many corn-sensitive patients who receive it would be exposed to the danger of severe reactions.

Invert sugar consists of fructose and dextrose derived from cane or beet sucrose. It is produced by heating the sucrose solution for a prolonged period in the presence of a weak acid.[28] Unfortunately, the fructose now widely used commercially is not the pure sugar but "high-fructose corn syrup."

SULFITES

In 1973, Kochen reported a case of recurrent asthma traced to the ingestion of dried fruits that had been treated with sulfur dioxide.[113] In cases since reported and in a discussion of five cases of their own, Stevenson and Simon found that most important sulfite to be potassium metabisulfite.[186] It is likely to be encountered in restaurants, where it is used as an antioxidant in potato dishes, salads, avocado dips, and wine.

SUNFLOWER SEED

Sunflower seed is roasted and eaten in the same manner as nuts. Allergy to sunflower seed is not rare and may be severe. This seed also is a source of an edible oil.

SURINAM CHERRY

This tropical fruit, also called pitanga, has a flavor described as tart, sweet, and slightly bitter.

SWEET POTATO

The sweet potato, the only plant of the morning glory family used as a food, rarely acts as an allergen. It is inclined, however, to cause gastrointestinal disturbances, especially in infants. Some of the soft, fleshy sweet potatoes are now called yams, but the true yam is an entirely unrelated plant.

SWISS CHARD

Like other members of the goosefoot family, Swiss chard seldom causes allergic reactions. In most parts of the country it grows well throughout the spring and summer.

TAMARIND

The pods of the tamarind tree contain a sweet pulp that is used in preserves, drinks, chutnies, and curries.

TAPIOCA

This starchy product has its origin in the rootstocks of cassava (manioc). It is used in puddings and fruit dishes, and its starch is useful as a substitute for wheat flour and corn starch in making cream sauces and gravies for patients allergic to wheat or corn. I have neither seen nor heard of tapioca acting as an allergen.

TARO

Taro is used in Hawaii chiefly in the form of poi, a paste made by boiling and grinding the roots and allowing them to ferment.

TARRAGON

This spice is used to make tarragon vinegar.

TEA

Green tea is obtained by drying the fresh leaves of the plant. Black or fermented tea is made from leaves that are first allowed to wilt and then rolled until the cell walls are broken. It is then allowed to ferment for several hours. Various spices are added to some types of tea, such as jasmine tea. Tea seldom acts as an allergen, but intolerance to its caffeine is common. Acceptable substitutes are the many so-called herb teas, consisting of a variety of herbs and spices. For example, Celestial Seasonings Lemon Mist herb tea contains lemon grass, lemon verbena, spearmint leaves, blackberry leaves, rose hips, comfrey leaves, lemon peel, orange blossoms, and orange peel.

THYME

This popular spice, like other mint spices, is an occasional allergen. It is used in clam chowder, meats, fish sauces, chipped beef, and fricassees. It goes well with fresh tomatoes.

TOMATO

The tomato is both a common food and a common allergen. It is an especially important cause of urticaria and eczema. Raw tomatoes are a common cause of aphthae (canker sores) and contact dermatitis of the hand.

TRAGACANTH

This leguminous shrub produces gum tragacanth, a thickening agent and stabilizer. It seems to be giving way to less expensive substitutes.

TRITICALE

This is a new grain, a hybrid of wheat and rice. It does not promise to be a popular food except, perhaps, among food faddists.

TRUFFLES

These are subterranean fungi highly prized by the gourmet and available only to the rich.

TURMERIC

In the United States, at least, this relative of ginger is used chiefly in the manufacture of cucumber pickles. It adds flavor and a yellow color. I have seen an occasional case of allergy to this spice.

TURNIP

Turnip is a hypoallergenic, nourishing, and inexpensive vegetable.

VANILLA

Vanilla is the contribution of the orchid family to the human dietary. The active principle, vanillin, is now produced synthetically.

VINEGAR

This word means sour wine, and wine vinegar is still the most delicious of the vinegars. In America apple cider vinegar has long been popular, but malt or distilled vinegar is rapidly taking its place.

Also used to some extent is pineapple vinegar. It represents what might be called the end process of beer manufacture. However, unlike apple vinegar, it does not seem to carry the antigenicity of the original product. Some patients insist that they do not tolerate vinegar of any kind, which suggests that the responsible allergen in such cases is acetic acid.

WALNUT

Black walnut and English walnut might be expected to cross-react closely, but they do not. Each is a common offender. Technically a walnut is a drupe (like a plum or almond), not a nut.

A nut closely related to black walnut is the butternut. It is apparently available commercially, but is gathered in rural areas from wild trees.

WATER CHESTNUT

This plant produces edible tubers which are regular constituents of many Chinese foods. It is a member of the sedge family and is not related to the true chestnut. It is interesting that a troublesome lawn weed, nut grass, a related plant, also produces edible tubers. They were a common food of the Indians.

WATERCRESS

This, another plant from the large mustard family, adds piquancy to salads.

WEST INDIAN CHERRY

This fruit is also known as Barbados or Puerto Rican cherry. It is sometimes confused with Surinam cherry.

WHEAT

Since wheat is such a basic food of the Western world, the patient who is sensitive to it has a difficult task of avoidance. The patient himself knows that he must pass up the market shelves displaying bread, cookies, crackers, and pastries. He also learns to avoid noodles, macaroni, spaghetti, pancakes, waffles, pretzels, wheat cereals, gravies, and cream sauces. More easily overlooked wheat-containing foods are certain types of chili and candies.

Wheat allergy is invariably severe and is inclined to cause an unusually large variety of allergic disorders. When a new patient comes in with "just about every complaint in the book" and appears to be seriously ill, I think immediately of allergy to wheat and its relatives.

WILD RICE

This member of the grass family is, like true rice, a water plant. Since it is such a gourmet food, I do not have enough experience with it to say whether it cross-reacts with the other grains, but I suspect it does.

WINTERGREEN

This flavoring agent was originally derived from various plants of the heath family, but synthetic wintergreen has replaced the natural product. My associates and I have documented one case of severe sensitivity to this spice and have since seen a milder case.[173] Wintergreen is used in root beer, candies, chewing gum, toothpastes, and liniments.

YAM

The yam is the large, fleshy, tuberous root of several species of *Dioscorea*. Yams are used as foods in the Pacific islands, northern Australia, and other tropical areas. Certain types of sweet potato are often called yams but they are totally unrelated to the true yam.

YEASTS

Various strains of yeast are essential to the baking of bread and the production of beer, wine, and other alcoholic beverages. Their prime function is the fermentation of sugars to produce alcohol and carbon dioxide, both of which are found in sparkling wines and beer. Whether or not there is enough yeast in baked goods and beverages to be allergenic is not clear. However, patients highly allergic to atmospheric molds seem to be made worse by unusually yeasty bread and beer.

Table 5-8
Food Names in English, French, Spanish, Italian, and German

English	French	Spanish	Italian	German
abalone	ormeau	oreja marina	crecchia marina	Seeohr
acorn	gland	bellota	ghianda	Eichel
allspice	pigment, toute épice	baya del pimiento de Jamaica	pimenti	Nelkenpfeffer
almond	amande	almendra	mandorla	Mandel
anchovy	anchoise	anchoa, boquerón	acciuga	Sardelle
apple	pomme	manzana	pomo	Apfel
apricot	abricot	albaricoque	albicocca	Aprikose
arrowroot	marante	arrurruz	maranta	Pfeilwurz
artichoke	artichaut	alcachofa	carciofo	Artischocke
asparagus	asperge	espárrago	asparago	Spargel
bacon	lard	tocino	lardo	Speck
banana	banane	plátano, banana	banana	Banane
barley	orge	cebada	orzo	Gerste, Graupen
basil	basilic	albahaca	basilico	Basileinkraut
bass	bar	perca, lobina	brauzino	Barsch
bay leaf	feuille laurier	hoja de lauro	lauro	Lorbeerblatt
bean	fève	haba, frijol	fava, fagiolo	Bohne
beef	viande de boeuf	carne de res	manzo	Rindfleisch
beer	bière	cerveza	birra	Bier
beet, beetroot	bette	remolacha, betabel	bietola	rote Rübe
blackberry	mûre sauvage	mora, zarza	mora selvatica	Brombeere
black pepper	poivre noir	pimienta negra	pepe	schwarzer Pfeffer
blueberry	airelle	arándano de color azul	murtillo	Blaubeere, Heidelbeere

English	French	Spanish	Italian	German
borage	bourrache	borraja	boragine	Borretsch
bran	son	afrecho, salvado	crusca	Kleie
Brazil nut	noix du Brésil	nuez de Brasil	noce del Brasile	Paranuss
breadfruit	fruit à pain	fruto de árbol del pan	albero del pane	Brotbaum
broad bean	fève de marais	haba	fava grande	Saubohne
broccoli	brocoli	brócoli	broccoli	Spargelkraut
Brussels sprouts	choux de Bruxelles	bretones, coles Bruselas	cavoli di Brusselle	Rosenkohl
buckwheat	sarrazin	trigo sarraceno	grano saraceno	Buchweisen
butter	beurre	mantequilla	burro	Butter
buttermilk	lait de beurre	suero de manteca	siero di latte	Buttermilch
cabbage	chou	repollo, col	cavolo	Kohl, Kraut
cantaloupe	melon cantaloup	melón de verano	mellone	Zuckermelone
cape gooseberry	alkénkenge	alquequenja	specie di fisolide	Stachelbeere
caper	câpre	alcaparra	cappero	Kaper
caraway	carvi	carvi	carvi, comino	Kümmel
carob bean	caroube	algarroba	carruba	Johannisbrot
carrot	carotte	zanahoria	carota	Mohrrübe, Karrote
cashew	noix de cajou	nuez de la India, anacardo	noce d'anacardo	Cachou
cassava	cassave	mandioca	tapioca, jucca	Kassaur
cauliflower	chou-fleur	coliflor	cavolofiore	Blumenkohl
celery	céleri	apio	sedano, apio	Zellerie
cheese	fromage	queso	cacio, formagio	Käse
cherry	cerise	cereza	ciliegia	Kirsch
chervil	cerfeuil	perifollo	certoglio	Kerbel

Table 5-8 *(continued)*

English	French	Spanish	Italian	German
chestnut	châtaigne	castaña	castagna	Kastanie
chicken	poulet	pollo	pollo, pulcino	Huhn
chickpea, garbanzo	pois chiche	garbanzo	cece	Kichererbse
chicory	chicorée	achicoria	cicoria	Zichorie
chives	ciboulette	cebolleta	cipollina	Schnittlauch
cider	cidre	sidra	sidro	Apfelsaft
cinnamon	cannelle	canela	cannella	Zimt, Kaneel
clam	peigne, palourde	almeja, peine	pettine	essbarre Muschel
clove	clou de girofle	clavo de olor	chiodo di garofano	Nelke
cockle	bucarde	coquina	tellina, cardio	Hertzmuschel
cod, codfish	morue	bacalao	merluzzo	Kabeljau, Dorsch
coriander	coriandre	cilantro	coriandolo	Koriander
corn, maize	maïs	maíz	granturco	Mais
cotton	coton	algodón	cotone	Baumwolle
crab	crabe	cangrejo, jaiba	granchio	Krabbe, Krebs
cranberry	airelle rouge	arándano	mortella di palude	Preiselbeere
cream	crème	crema, nata	panna	Sahne, Rahm
cucumber	concombre	pepino	cetriolo	Gurke
currant	groseille rouge	grosella	ribes	Johannesbeere
curry	curry	curry, cari	condire all'Indiana	Curry, indisches Ragoutpulver
custard	flan, crème	flan, natillas	crema carmella	Eierrahm
dill	aneth	eneldo	aneto	Dill
duck	canard	pato, ánade	anitra	Ente

English	French	Spanish	Italian	German
eel	anguille	ánguila	anguilla	Aal
egg	oeuf	huevo	uovo	Ei
eggplant	aubergine	berenjena	melanzana	Aubergine
elderberry	baie de sureau	baya de saúco	sambuco	Holunderbeere
endive	endive	endibia	indivia	Endive
fennel	fennouil	hinojo	finocchio	Fenchel
fenugreek	fenugrec	fenogreco	fieno greco	Bockshorn Kraut
fig	figue	higo	fico	Feige
filbert, hazelnut	aveline	avellana	avellana	Haselnuss
flounder	flet	lenguado	passerino	Flunder
flour	farine	harina	farina	Mehl
frog	grenouille	rana	rana	Frosch
garlic	ail	ajo	aglio	Knoblauch
ginger	gingembre	gengibre	zenzero	Ingwer, Gember
goat	chèvre	cabra, chiva	capra	Ziege
goose	oie	ganso	oca, papera	Gans
gooseberry	groseille á maquereau	uva espina	uva spina, ribes	Stachelbeere
granadilla	grenadille	granadilla	granadiglia	Passionfrucht
grape	raisin	uva	uva	Weinbeere, Traube
grapefruit	pamplemousse	toronja	pompelmo	Pampelmuse
guava	goyave	guayaba	guaiva	Guajabe
haddock	aiglefin	besugo, róbalo	merluzzo	Schellfisch
halibut	flétan	mero, cherna	grosso rombo	Heilbutt
ham	jambon	jamón	prosciutto	Schinken

Table 5-8 (*continued*)

English	French	Spanish	Italian	German
hare, rabbit (US)	lièvre	liebre	lepre	Hase
hen	poule	gallina	gallina, chioccia	Henne, Huhn
herring	hareng	arenque	aringa	Hering
honey	miel	miel	miele	Honig
hop	houblon	lúpulo	luppulo	Hopfen
horseradish	raifort	rábano silvestre	rafano	Heerrettich
ice cream	glace	helado	gelato	Speiseeis
Jerusalem artichoke	topinambour	cotufa, ajipa, pataca	topinambur	Erdartischoke
kale	chou frisé	bretón	cavolo	Grünkohl, Winterkohl
kid	chevreau	cabrito	capretto	Zicklein
kohlrabi	chou-rave	colirrábano	cavolrapa	Kohlrabi
lamb	agneau	cordero	agnello	Lamm
leek	poireau	puerro	porro	Lauch
lemon	citron, limon	limón	limone	Zitrone
lentil	lentille	lenteja	lenticchia	Linse
lettuce	laitue	lechuga	lattuga	Lattach, Kopfsalat
licorice	réglisse	regaliz, alcazuz	liquirizia	Lakritze, Sussholz
lime	lime	lima	cedro, lima	Limone
liver	foie	hígado	fegato	Leber
lobster	homard	langosta de mar	aragosta	Hummer, Seekrebs
mace	macis	macia	macia	Musdelblüte
mackerel	maquereau	escombro	sgombro	Makrele
maple	érable	arce	acero	Ahorn
majoram	marjolaine	mejorana, orégano	maggiorana	Majoran

English	French	Spanish	Italian	German
milk	lait	leche	latte	Milch
mulberry	mûre	mora	mora, gelsa mora	Maulbeere
mushroom	champignon	seta, hongo	fungo, mangereccio	essbarer Pilz
mussel	moule	almeja	dattero di mare	Miesmuschel
mustard	moutarde	mostaza	senape, mostarda	Senf
mutton	mouton	carne de cordero	montone	Hammelfleisch
noodles	nouilles	pasta, tallarín	tagliatelli, pasta	Nudeln
nutmeg	muscade	nuez moscada	noce moscata	Muskatnuss
oats	avoine	avena	avena	Hafer
octopus	pieuvre	pulpo	ottopode, polpo	Oktopus
okra, gumbo	gombo, gobo	quimbombo	ibisco	Eibisch
olive	olive	aceituna	oliva	Olive
onion	oignon	cebolla	cipolla	Zwiebel
orange	orange	naranja	arancia	Orange, Apfelsine
oyster	huitre	ostra	ostrica	Auster
papaya, paw-paw (Brit)	papaye	papaya	papaia	Melonenbaum
parsley	persil	perejil	prezzemolo	Petersilie
parsnip	panais	chirivía	pastinaca	Pastinak
peach	pêche	melocotón, durazno	pesca	Pfirsich
peanut (groundnut)	arachide, cacahuète	cacahuate, maní	arachide, pistachio di terra	Erdnuss
pear	poire	pera	pera	Birne
peas (green)	petits pois	guisantes, chícharos	verdi piselli	kleine Erbse

150

Table 5-8 *(continued)*

English	French	Spanish	Italian	German
pecan	pécan	nuez de nogal americana	noce d'America	Hickorynuss
pepper (red, cayenne)	poivre de cayenne	pimienta de cayena	pepe di Caienna	Cayennepfeffer, Paprika
peppermint	menthe poivrée	hierbabuena, menta	menta peperina	Pfefferminze
perch	perche	perca	pesce persico	Barsch
persimmon	plaquemine	fruta de diáspiro	luccio	Dattelpflaume
pineapple	ananas	piña, anana	ananas	Ananas
plum	prune	ciruela	prugna, susina	Pflaume
pomegranate	grenade	granada	melgrana	Granatapfel
pork	viande de porc	carne de puerco	carne di maiale	Schweinefleisch
potato	pomme de terre	papa, patata	patata	Kartoffel
pumpkin	citrouille	calabaza	zucca, popone	Kürbis
purslane	pourpier	verdolaga	portulaca	Portulak
quince	coing	menbrilla	cotogna	Quitte
rabbit	lapin	conejo	coniglio	Kaninchen
radish	radis	rábano	ramolaccio	Rettich
raisin	raisin sec	pasa	uva secca	Rosine
rape	colza	nabo silvestre	colza	Raps
raspberry	framboise	frambuesa	lampone	Himbeere
rhubarb	rhubarbe	ruibarbo	rabarbaro	Rhabarber
rice	riz	arroz	riso	Reis
rutabaga, swede	suedoise	naba de Suecia	rapa suedese	Kohlrübe
rye	seigle	centeno	segale	Roggen
sage	sauge	salvia	salvia	Salbei
salad	salade	ensalada	insalata	Salat

English	French	Spanish	Italian	German
salmon	saumon	salmón	salmone	Lachs
salsify, oyster plant	salsifis	salsifí	sassefrica	Haferwurz, Bocksbart
sauerkraut	choucroute	chocruta	salcraratte	Sauerkraut
sausage	saucisse	chorizo, salchichón	salciccia	Wurst
savory	sarriette	ajedrea	savore	Bohnenkraut
scallop	pétoncle	venera	petonchio	Kammuschel
seaweed	algue marine	alga marina	alga	Alge
sesame	sésame	ajonjolí	sesamo	Sesam
shad	alose	alosa	alosa	Alse
shallot	échalotte	escalona, chalote	scalogno	Schallotte
shark	requin	tiburón	squalo	Hai
shrimp	crevette	camarón, gamba	gamberetto	Garnele
snail	escargot	caracol	chiocciola	Schnecke
sole	sole	lenguado	sogliola	Seezunge
spinach	épinard	espinaca	spinagio	Spinat
sprat	esprot	sardineta	spratto	Sprotte
squash, marrow	courgette	calabaza	zucca	Kürbis
squid	calmar	calamar	calamaro, seppia	Tintenfisch
strawberry	fraise	fresa, frutillo	fragola	Erdbeere
sugar	sucre	azúcar	zucchero	Zucker
sugarcane	canne à sucre	caña de azúcar	canna de zucchero	Zuckerrohr
sunflower	tournesol	girasol	girasole	Sonnenblume
sweet potato	patate	batata, camote	patata dolce	Batate
tamarind	tamarin	tamarindo	tamarindo	Tamarinde

Table 5-8 (*continued*)

English	French	Spanish	Italian	German
tapioca	tapioca	mandioca, tapioca	tapioca	Tapioca
tea	thé	té	tè	Tee
thyme	thym	tomillo	timo	Thymian
trout	truite	trucha	trota	Forelle
tuna fish, tunny	thun	atún	tonno	Thunfisch
turkey	dindon	guajalote, pavo	tacchino	Truthahn
turmeric	curcume	cúrcuma	curcuma	Gelbwurz
turnip, neep	navet	nabo	rapa	Steckrübe
venison	venaison	carne de venado	cervo	Hirsch
vinegar	vinaigre	vinagre	aceto	Essig
walnut	noix	nuez de nogal	noce	Walnuss
watercress	cresson de fontaine	berro de agua	crescione	Brunnenkresse
watermelon	melon d'eau	sandía	cocomero	Wassermelone
wheat	froment, blé	trigo	frumento	Weizen
wintergreen	pyrole	pirola	gaulteria	Wintergrün
yam (true)*	igname	ñame	igname	Samswurzel
yeast	levure, ferment	levadura	lievito	Hefe

*Sweet potato is often falsely known as yam.

In this table are listed the common names of foods as they occur in the major languages of the Western World. Whenever the native language of the physician is not the same as that of the patient, this table can make for more satisfactory communication. I have found this especially true in talking with patients whose native language is Spanish, many of whom are to be found in the United States.

Not listed in the table are foods that are the same, or virtually so, in all of these languages. Examples are agar, anise, annatto, avocado, bamboo, cardamom, carp, chicle, chocolate, cochineal, coconut, coffee, cola, cumin, date, gelatine, guar, gum, karaya, kumquat, macaroni, mango, mayonnaise, melon, mint, pistachio, saffron, sago, sardine, sesame, soy, spaghetti, tomato, and vanilla.

6 • DETECTION OF FOOD ALLERGENS

Foods are seldom the only factors affecting the allergic patient. Inhalant allergy is almost always present, and the possibility of contact and drug allergy must often be considered. To further complicate the situation, factors other than allergy may also be present. For these reasons, all but the simplest cases of food allergy call for a complete allergy workup.

In this chapter we will discuss the part of the allergy workup that is devoted to the detection of food allergens. We will begin with a review of the essentials of this clinical procedure.

THE ESSENTIALS OF FOOD DETECTION

Knowledge of Manifestations

Someone has compared allergic patients to a population of guinea pigs who have been sensitized to various antigens and then turned loose without identification. If we continue the analogy, the allergist may be compared to the person charged with determining to which antigens each guinea pig is sensitive. Allergy practice is, of course, much more complicated than this: sensitized guinea pigs react in a predictable fashion, while allergic patients react in a bewildering variety of ways. The allergist must therefore know not only the many *causes* of allergy but its many *manifestations.* These have been discussed in Chapter 3.

It is important that minor manifestations are not neglected. The reason for this is that such major allergic disorders as asthma, urticaria, eczema, and migraine tend to flare periodically, while such minor symptoms as increased throat mucus and gastrointestinal distress are inclined to be constant. Finding the cause of minor complaints is therefore important in that it often reveals the cause of the major complaints. In discussing this with patients I explain that we proceed much like a district attorney investigating a gang leader—the investigation doesn't begin with the leader but with the petty hoodlums under his command.

Differential Diagnosis

Since food allergy is usually a systemic disorder, we must be constantly on the alert not to overlook nonallergic diseases, some of which may be serious. This is especially important if the patient comes in of his own volition (as is so often the case) rather than by referral. Whenever there is doubt, I ask the patient to check possible nonallergic factors with his own physician.

Differential diagnosis also includes consideration of allergens other than foods. *Inhalants* are, after all, more important than foods and may cause similar symptoms. They may play a role not only in respiratory tract allergy but in eczema, urticaria, and headache. The number of *drugs* capable of acting as allergens is unlimited; the most likely to cause chronic, obscure symptoms are aspirin,[183] diuretics, laxatives, and anticonvulsants, but any drug the patient takes should be under some suspicion. In eczema, such *contactants* as nickel, neomycin, plants, artificial rubber, and paraben preservatives must also be considered.

Knowledge of Food Relationships

I recently saw a patient who reported that she could not eat foods containing rosemary or thyme and invariably became ill after eating lamb. Since rosemary and thyme are members of the mint family, I suspected that mint jelly served with lamb might be the offender rather than the lamb itself. This proved to be the case. Thus knowledge of the relationships of foods, especially those of plant origin, is helpful in the identification of food allergens. (See Chapter 4.) The relationship of common foods is outlined in Table 6-1.

Table 6-1
Abbreviated Food Family List

	Plant Families
Apple	apple
Banana	banana
Buckwheat	buckwheat, rhubarb
Cashew	cashew, pistachio, mango
Citrus	orange, lemon, grapefruit
Cola	chocolate, cola
Fungi	yeast, mushroom
Ginger	ginger, turmeric
Goosefoot	beet, spinach

Table 6-1 *(continued)*

Gourd	cucumber, pumpkin, melons, squash
Grape	grape
Grass	corn, wheat, rice, oats, barley, rye
Heath	blueberry, cranberry
Laurel	cinnamon, bay leaf, avocado
Lily	onion, garlic, asparagus
Madder	coffee
Mallow	okra, cottonseed
Mint	mint, thyme, sage
Morning glory	sweet potato
Mustard	mustard, cabbage, cauliflower, broccoli, Brussels sprouts, turnip, radish, horseradish
Myrtle	allspice, clove
Nightshade	tomato, potato, eggplant, peppers
Olive	olive
Palm	coconut, date
Parsley	carrot, celery, cumin, coriander
Pea	pea, peanut, beans, soybean
Pepper	black (and white) pepper
Pineapple	pineapple
Plum	almond, plum, peach, cherry, apricot
Rose	strawberry, raspberry, blackberry
Sunflower	lettuce, sunflower seed
Tea	tea

Animal Classification

Mollusks	Oster, clam, scallop, cockle, snail, octopus, squid
Crustaceans	Shrimp, lobster, crab
Fish	Shark, herring, carp, tarpon, cod, haddock, perch, flounder, halibut, trout, salmon, tuna, mackerel, catfish, sole, anchovy
Amphibia	Frog
Reptiles	Turtle
Birds	Chicken, turkey, duck, goose, eggs
Mammals	Beef, pork, lamb, cow and goat milk

Familiarity with Individual Foods

Just as the bacteriologist must be an expert on bacteria and other microorganisms, the allergist must be an expert on foods. He must be familiar with their appearance, availability, digestibility, nutritional value, and flavor, and he must know how they appear in the dietary. When going through a cafeteria line with trainees whose English is not fluent, I insist they tell the waitress the name of each food and not simply point a finger at it. It is absolutely necessary that the allergist know foods. Otherwise he cannot give intelligent advice to patients on food avoidance and food substitution.

Knowing which Food Allergens are Most Common

It is often said that the most common food allergens are fish, nuts, and chocolate. If we rephrase this to read, "The most *obvious* food allergens are fish, nuts, and chocolate," we are nearer the truth. The common *allergens* are, in fact, the common *foods,* those eaten daily or almost daily. Table 6-2 summarizes the findings of four separate studies. It shows that the ten most common offenders are as follows (the percentage represents incidence of allergic reaction in patients known to have food allergy):

Milk	65%
Chocolate, cola	45%
Corn	30%
Legumes, egg	26%
Citrus	25%
Tomato	16%
Wheat, rice	11%
Pork	10%
Cinnamon	8%

Since milk allergy occurs in well over half of patients who are allergic to foods, it is obvious that it should be investigated in virtually every case. As early as 1888 Hopkins, an Englishman, placed milk first in the list of foods likely to cause "idiosyncrasy."[95] It is also listed in first place by Blue of the United States[19] and Solari of Argentina.[170] When the incidence of milk allergy was compared with the incidence of allergy to other foods, four observers found milk allergy to be the most common. They are Kaplan of South Africa (34 of 49 cases, 70%),[105] Sethi et al of India (14 of 41 cases, 34%),[164] Mackie of the United States (26 of 33 cases, 79%),[126] and Nogaller and Gorbunof of Russia (233 of 418 cases, 56%).[140]

Ranking next after the allergens listed in Table 6-2 are fish, potato, onion, apple, beef, crustaceans (especially shrimp), artificial food colors, black pepper, and banana.

Table 6-2
The Ten Common Food Allergens

Type of Patient	No.	Milk	Choc. Cola	Corn	Leg- umes	Egg	Citrus	Tomato	Wheat Rice	Pork	Cin- namon
Children[177]	514	321	241	152	117	145	115	64	55	18	51
Headache[178]	98	83	44	34	25	14	13	--	9	23	13
Multiple Foods[182]	250	185	118	88	98	72	98	72	34	46	--
ASA-sensitive[183]	112	44	34	16	15	20	19	17	8	11	11
Total	974	633	437	290	255	251	245	153	106	98	75
Percentage		65	45	30	26	26	25	16	11	10	8

In these studies chocolate and cola were found to cross-react very closely, citrus fruits somewhat less so, and legumes (peanut, soybean, common bean, pea, etc.) least of all. Almost all patients sensitive to wheat were sensitive to rice and vice versa.

The Allergy History

Like any other medical history, the allergy history covers all factors, allergic or otherwise, that may be related to the patient's state of health. Among the nonallergic factors to be considered are all the important diseases the patient has (or has had), any surgical procedures that have been performed, and any drugs that have been taken or are being taken.

The part of the history dealing specifically with allergy is made up of two distinct parts. The first is a review of all symptoms that may be of allergic origin. The second is a search for clues as to responsible inhalants, foods, drugs, contactants, and injectants. Also included is an investigation of such nonspecific factors as odors, fumes, infection, chilling, overheating, and emotional and physical stress.

Skin Testing

The number of skin tests used in a workup depends on the allergens to which the patient is likely to be exposed. This differs greatly from one part of the world to another. Although skin tests are of marginal value in food allergy, the allergist who does not use them deprives himself of help in a situation in which he needs all the help he can get. No one has expressed this better than Blue: "Even though these tests have shortcomings in a high percentage of instances, this is no reason to disregard them. . . . By weighing the elements of error or false-positive tests and by carefully coordinating this finding with a careful history, much helpful information can be gained."[19]

An interesting point made by Osvath et al[145] is that milk-sensitive patients tend strongly to have positive skin tests to cattle hair. I have found that they also tend to react on skin test to beef without necessarily proving to be allergic to beef.

Figure 6-1 is a condensed version of the form used in our clinic. It lists both the inhalant and food allergens which are tested. Inhalants are checked by punch or scratch tests and if negative, the important offenders are checked by intradermal tests. Foods are checked by punch or scratch tests only.

ELIMINATION DIET

The history taken at the first visit will usually indicate whether or not the patient's complaints are related to foods. It may also provide clues as to responsible offenders.

When the history places certain foods under suspicion, these and

Figure 6-1

NASAL	Block	Discharge	Sneeze	Throat-Mucus	Epistaxis	Rept URI

CHEST	Cough	Dyspnea	Wheezing	Mucus	Rept-Bronchitis/Pneumonia

EAR	EYE	HEADACHE	TENSION	FATIGUE	ACHING

INSECT STINGS	G.I. Pain	Constipation	Diarrhea	Distension	Aphthae

ECZEMA CONTACT DERM. URTICARIA/AG.EDEMA NONALLERGIC ILLS, SURGERY

PILLOW MATTRESS HOUSE PETS Jan Feb Mar Apr May Jun Jly Aug Sep Oct Nov Dec

OCCUPATION	HOUSE	X-RAY	LAB

SUSPECTS	SCRATCH TESTS		INTRADERMAL
Inhalants	Alternaria	Aspergillus	TESTS
	Hormodendrum	Helminthosporium	
	Spondylocladium	House Dust	
	Phoma	Ragweed Mix	
	Monilia sitophila	Burweed Marsh Elder	
	Fusarium	Brewer's Yeast	
			ELIMINATION
	Kochia	Blue Grass	DIETS
	Russian Thistle	Bermuda Grass	
	Water Hemp	Meadow Fescue Grass	
	Mixed Feathers	Brome Grass	
	Cat Hair	Tobacco	
Foods	Dog Hair	Cottonseed	
	Elm	Guinea Pig	
	Red Oak	Hamster	
	Maple	Rabbit	
	Cattle Hair	Jute	
	Horse Hair	Wool	
	Pyrethrum	Linters	
	Almond	Cashew Nut	
	Beef	Chocolate	
	Black Pepper	Cinnamon	PATCH TESTS
Drugs	Brazil Nut	Coconut	
	Buckwheat	Egg	
	Carrot	Grape	
	Hazelnut	Shrimp	
	Milk	Soybean	
	Mustard	Tomato	
	Peanut	Tuna Fish	
	Peppermint	Walnut	
	Pork	Wheat	

related products should be eliminated. If there are no clues, I defer the elimination diet study until a second visit a week or so later. An accurate allergy history is difficult to obtain, and the patient will be in a better position to cooperate after having time to think about his case. During the four or five visits we set aside for the workup, skin tests for foods are done. I am careful to explain that they are used mainly to pick up an occasional "sleeper" that might be missed in the elimination diet studies. I also explain that final determination of the role of foods as allergens depends on elimination and challenge, not skin tests.

Table 6-3 shows the elimination diet form used in our clinic. It consists of two parts. The first is a list of the ways common food allergens appear in the dietary. The symptoms under investigation are underlined for the specific patient, and any not printed on the form are added. The second part is a list of the constituents of common foods. The foods to be eliminated are circled and the number of days of avoidance noted. The patient is instructed to watch for relief of the indicated symptoms.

Table 6-3
Elimination Diet

	ELIMINATE FOODS CIRCLED BELOW FOR THE NUMBER OF DAYS SHOWN. Watch for relief of the following symptoms: nasal congestion, cough, chest/throat mucus, wheezing, constipation, diarrhea, stomach ache, bloating, poor appetite, eczema, hives, headache, tension, fatigue, breath odor, sweating.
_____days	1. MILK (dried, 2%, evaporated, skim, buttermilk). Sherbet, ice cream, yogurt, custard, creamed foods. Cheese. (slight traces of milk OK)
_____days	2. CHOCOLATE and COLA (Coca-Cola, Pepsi, RC, Tab, Diet Rite, etc.)
_____days	3. CORN.* *Corn syrup* (sweetener): candy, catsup, sweetened cereals, most baked goods (bread, buns, cookies, cake), canned fruits and juices, jelly, gum, prepared meats (hot dogs, sausage, lunch ham), ice cream, carbonated drinks, Kool-Aid, peanut butter, pancake syrup. *Cornstarch:* soups, gravies, powdered sugar. *Cornmeal:* baked goods, fish sticks and chips, Mexican foods (tacos, tamales, Fritos, etc.), Corn Curls, popcorn, Cracker Jacks, hominy, grits, corn on cob, canned corn, whiskey (bourbon, Canadian), beer. *Corn flour. Corn oil, Corn oil margarines. Corn cereals.*

These foods do *not* contain corn.* Corn-free baked goods, mayonnaise, sugar, brown sugar, honey, spices. Cottonseed,

Table 6-3 *(continued)*

soy, olive, and safflower oils. Spry, Crisco, lard, butter, most margarines. Any vegetable but corn, salads, fruits (fresh, dried, home-canned with sugar, dietetic). Ham, bacon, fresh meat, fish, chicken, turkey, shrimp, oysters. Olives, potato chips, french fries, pickles, peanuts, other nuts. Soda pop, coffee, tea, pure sugar candy, macaroni, spaghetti, noodles, pretzels. Wine, scotch, vodka, gin, brandy. Egg. Milk, cheese. No list of corn syrup sources is ever complete, and the way it is used throughout the world varies greatly from place to place.

_____days 4. EGG.* Baked goods (*except* simple bread, cookies, crackers), pancakes, waffles, noodles, mayonnaise, creamy salad dressings, meat loaf, breaded foods, meringue, custard, french toast, divinity, icings.

_____days 5. PEA FAMILY. Beans, peas, peanuts, peanut butter, peanut oil, soybean,* chili, honey. (Watch for soy oil and flour, now widely used!)

_____days 6. CITRUS. Orange, lemon, lime, tangerine, grapefruit (and their juices).

_____days 7. TOMATO. Juice, paste, salads, pizza, chili, catsup, steak sauce, soups, stews, tacos, and many mixed dishes such as Italian foods.

_____days 8. SMALL GRAINS (wheat most important). WHEAT, RICE, BARLEY, OATS. Wheat* is used in all breads (including rye and corn), rolls, cakes, cookies, crackers, doughnuts, pie crust, waffles, pancakes, pretzels, ice cream cones, macaroni, spaghetti, noodles, gravy, chili, cream sauce. Small grains are used in breakfast cereals and beer. Some patients must also avoid RYE.

_____days 9. CINNAMON.* Widely used in spice cakes, cookies, rolls, pies, candy, apple dishes, gum, catsup, chili, hot dogs and other prepared meats.

_____days 10. PORK. Fresh pork, ham, bacon, ground meats (lunch ham, spreads, wieners, frankfurters, sausage, etc), lard.

*All the ways that corn, egg, soybean, wheat, and cinnamon are used may not be listed here. The patient needs to check ingredients himself.

There are two methods of selecting foods for elimination. The first depends on the history and, occasionally, on skin test reactions. When, for example, there is evidence against wheat, peanut, and egg, the foods to be eliminated are the small grains, the legumes (pea family), and egg. The second method is used when there are no clues. On the basis of probabilities, the top three offenders, milk, chocolate/cola, and corn, are eliminated. In serious cases calling for prompt action, severe asthma for example, all ten common groups of foods shown in Table 6-2 are eliminated at the same time. This may be called the "multiple exclusion diet."

After elimination comes challenge, the returning of the foods being tested. The first food is returned after ten days. Thereafter, at 2- to 4-day intervals, the other foods are returned one at a time. With the return of each food, the patient or (in the case of a child) the parents watch for a return of the symptoms being studied.

When there is a clear-cut history of severe allergy to a food, challenge is unnecessary and may be dangerous. This is especially true in infants and children.[67] Just as no physician will challenge a patient with a drug that has obviously caused a severe adverse reaction neither should he do so with a food with such a history. Theoretically challenge should be "double-blind," but as Tolber points out, this is not clinically practical.[193]

It is sometimes helpful to have the patient keep a diet diary. He is given a form with seven horizontal columns, one for each day of the week, and four vertical columns, for listing foods eaten at breakfast, lunch, and supper. Snacks are entered in the column of the closest meal; drugs taken are entered in the same way. Symptoms with their time of occurrence are listed in the fourth column. By studying the patient's notes the physician can sometimes establish a cause-and-effect relationship between foods and manifestations. This is more likely to prove true in urticaria than in other allergic disorders.

When the patient on the multiple exclusion diet discovers that all common foods are excluded, his natural reaction is to ask what he *can* eat. Except for any that are under suspicion, the following foods are allowed:

Vegetables and salads: artichoke, asparagus, avocado, beet, broccoli, buckwheat, carrot, cauliflower, celery, Chinese cabbage, chives, collards, cucumber, kohlrabi, lettuce, mushroom, okra, onion, parsnip, peppers, potato, radish, rhubarb, rutabaga, spinach, squash (summer and winter), sweet potato, turnip, and water chestnut.

Starches: arrowroot, tapioca, and potato.

Fruits: apple, apricot, banana, blueberry, boysenberry, cantaloupe, cherry, cranberry, date, fig, gooseberry, grape (and grape juice, raisins, and wine), mango, nectarine, papaya, peach, pear, pineapple and pineapple juice, plum and prune, pumpkin, raspberry, strawberry, and watermelon. (No fruits canned in syrup are to be used.)

Spices and herbs: allspice, clove, comino, coriander, ginger, horseradish, mace, marjoram, mint, mustard, nutmeg, oregano, paprika, red pepper, sage, and thyme.

Sugars: beet, cane, and maple.

Oils: coconut, cottonseed, olive, and safflower.

Miscellaneous: olive, vinegar, salt, tea, and uncolored, noncola carbonated drinks.

Meats: beef, lamb, chicken, turkey, fish, oyster, shrimp. (If the patient is allergic to these foods—beef excepted—he will know it. This may not be true, however, of children.)

On one occasion while I was explaining the elimination diet to the mother of a high-school boy, he remarked, "Doctor, I don't think this is a very well-controlled test." He pointed out that while foods were being checked, other means of relieving his symptoms, inhalant control and hyposensitization, for example, were being carried out. I had, of course, to agree with him. But I also pointed out that prompt relief of his illness called for proceeding at once with all methods at our disposal. Some allergists prefer to defer elimination diet study until inhalant factors, if present, are worked out. This is perhaps the best way to proceed in cases mild enough to allow such a leisurely process.

REACTIONS TO DRUGS

As we have seen, food allergy greatly resembles drug allergy. In both types the diagnosis is by clinical methods, and the treatment is simple avoidance. It is important to note that drug allergy is especially common in patients with multiple food and inhalant allergy. It is more likely to occur in women than in men and children.

Identification of drug allergens depends on a history directed specifically toward drugs. Since it may occur in any patient, allergic or otherwise, every patient is questioned carefully. He is asked to list all drugs he is taking or has taken. To aid his memory, inquiry is made as to the following common drugs and classes of drugs: Aarane, acetaminophen, aerosols, allergy injections, analgesics, antibiotics, anticoagulants, antidepressants, antifungal drugs, antihistamines, aspirin, asthma medicines, beclomethazone, Butazolidine, codeine, cold tablets, cough medicines, cromolyn, Darvon, Datril, decongestants, digitalis, diuretics, ephedrine, ergotamine, erythromycin, Fiorinal, Furadantin, Gynergen, headache remedies, hydantoins, Indocin, indomethacin, Intal, laxatives, lozenges, Macrodantin, methylphenidate, methysergide, muscle relaxants, nitrofurantoin, nose drops and sprays, oral contraceptives, Orinase, penicillin, pentazocine, phenothiazines, phenylbutazone, phenylpropanolamine, Propadrine, propoxyphene, propranolol, quinine (in "tonic"), rectal medications, Ritalin, Sansert, sulfonamides, Talwin, terbutaline, tetracyclines, theophylline, tolbutamide, tranquilizers, Tylenol, vaginal medications, Vanceril.

Drug allergy is a complex problem and one too extensive for further consideration here. The physician will find *AMA Drug Evaluations* of tremendous aid, not only in checking for drug reactions but for drug indications. Also of value are the *Physicians' Desk Reference* (PDR) and package inserts. In unusual cases, textbooks devoted exclusively to drug reactions may be consulted.

7 • TREATMENT OF FOOD ALLERGY

Once a case of food allergy has been worked out, management depends chiefly on avoidance of the offending allergens. It is therefore necessary that patients understand how the foods they are allergic to may appear in the diet. This information is given in Table 6-3, Chapter 6.

Avoidance does not always need to be absolute. In many cases allergy to foods is variable, depending on fluctuations in the patient's tolerance. An understanding of tolerance is therefore important in the management of food allergy.[153,157]

TOLERANCE

The adverse reaction caused by an allergen is often uniform, predictable, and absolute. This is *fixed sensitivity*, a state of permanent intolerance. It is the characteristic response to drugs and to such potent inhalants as horse and cat epithelials. Some patients are so sensitive to foods they even react to food odors. Gould and Pyle report many cases from as early as the sixteenth century of patients being made ill by the odors of apple, cherry, bread, cheese, cinnamon, and sassafras.[77] In 1893 Raymond wrote:

> I was told by Professor Walter S. Haines of a clergyman in an eastern city who, being the unhappy possessor of this peculiarity, was forced to request friends with whom he would dine to allow no raw apples to be put on the table else he would succumb to the ill effects of their odor, which effect was a most distressing illness.[152]

In 1917 Frost reported:

> I would just like to speak of a peculiar instance of a food idiosyncrasy occurring in a family which in each of three generations showed this idiosyncrasy. Thinking it might be merely imagination, someone tried putting onions near one of these individuals while he was asleep, and as a result he was sick for a week.[70]

Many other cases of allergy to food odors have been reported in the literature.[1,31,46,52,60,62,96,197]

Fixed sensitivity to foods is especially common in allergy to fish,

165

cinnamon, artificial food colors, and shrimp. It is also common in allergy to seeds used as *grains* (corn and buckwheat, *nuts* (peanut and Brazil nut), *spices* (black pepper and mustard), and *beverages* (chocolate and coffee). Patients with this type of sensitivity soon learn the necessity of complete avoidance.

When sensitivity fluctuates in response to either host factors or environmental influences, it is known as *variable sensitivity*. Foods to which there may be variable sensitivity include milk, egg, pork, beef, potato, tomato, citrus fruits, onion, cabbage, and tea. It will be noted that none of these foods is derived from seeds. The patient with variable sensitivity to a food tends to gain tolerance when conditions are favorable and to lose it when they are not.

Factors that Lower Tolerance

Infection   Although tolerance may be lowered by almost anything that has an adverse effect on the patient, infection is by far the most important. This applies especially to respiratory allergy but also, to some extent at least, to eczema and gastrointestinal allergy. The fact that both parents and physicians tend to keep milk away from sick children is probably based on the fact that many children with variable tolerance to milk lose it when ill. Everyone has heard the comments, "Milk thickens mucus" and "Starve a cold."

Cold   Food allergy should always be suspected when the patient is worse in the winter. This is partly because this is the season when respiratory infections are common, but it also depends on the fact that the patient who is chilled tends to lose tolerance to both foods and inhalants. Many patients remark, "I am allergic to cold and drafts."

Heavy inhalant load   During times of the year when the atmosphere is heavily polluted with pollens and molds, many patients learn to be especially careful to avoid foods they can ordinarily eat with little, if any, trouble. Patients allergic to ragweed pollen may find that certain raw fruits and vegetables make them worse at the peak of the season. We may speculate that these foods are histamine releasers, but scientific evidence is scanty. Common offenders are melons, orange, lettuce, tomato, carrots, and celery.

Degree and frequency of exposure   Many egg-sensitive patients notice no reaction whatever if they eat an egg occasionally, at intervals, perhaps, of five or six days. They may also be able to tolerate such traces as are found in noodles and cake. Almost all milk-sensitive patients can ignore traces of milk in bread and butter and many can have a small amount of milk, cheese, or ice cream once a week. There is always the danger, however, that such patients may decide they are outgrowing a sensitivity of this type and return to their former intake.

Humidity   Rowe has pointed out that the patient who must carefully watch his diet in damp areas and during damp seasons can be much less strict in the desert or during periods of drought.[157] When stationed in the South Pacific, I found it necessary to evacuate several young men from the Solomon Islands because of asthma apparently brought on by the constant high humidity characteristic of that part of the world.

Other stress   It may be said that virtually anything that has an adverse effect on the food-sensitive patient tends to lower tolerance. Examples are fatigue, emotional stress, and intercurrent organic disease.

Factors that Raise Tolerance

In general, the things that raise tolerance are the direct opposite of those that lower it. Patients usually have more tolerance in hot, dry weather, when free of infection, and when the level of airborne pollens and molds is low. Hyposensitization to pollens, molds, and house dust may eventually bring about complete tolerance. On a temporary basis, adrenal corticosteroids have the same effect.

To some extent, variable tolerance is raised by abstinence. This is especially true of milk allergy. A patient who has avoided milk and milk products completely for a month or so may find that he can have them in moderate amounts. Unfortunately, he often exceeds his tolerance without knowing it and must be cautioned to limit his milk intake.

FOOD AVOIDANCE IN THE VARIOUS ALLERGIC DISORDERS

Only occasionally are allergic diseases caused by food allergy alone. When they are, of course, the only treatment necessary is avoidance in conformity with the patient's tolerance. But in the average case, other causes, both allergic and nonallergic, must be kept in mind. We will now consider, necessarily in outline form, some of the factors to be considered in the various disorders that may be associated with food allergy.

Headache

Few manifestations may be caused by a wider variety of factors than headache. Before allergy study is undertaken it is therefore essential that other, perhaps more serious, causes be investigated. When this has been accomplished and the headache appears to be functional, not only food allergy but inhalant allergy should be considered. Other possible precipitants of attacks are odors and fumes, premenstrual tension, psychic and physical stress, oral contraceptives, chilling, caffeine, and alcohol.[181]

Gastrointestinal Allergy

The fact that foods "disagree" with an individual does not necessarily mean that the problem is food allergy. Any underlying organic disease may be activated by foods that are not easily digested. Examples are hiatal hernia, peptic ulcer, gall bladder disease, and various diseases of the colon. Examples of foods that are not easily digested are cabbage, onion, radish, apple, cashew nut, melons, black pepper, coconut, beans, banana, coffee, pineapple, and pork.

Pruritus Ani

Although food allergy often causes this tormenting problem, almost any disorder of the lower intestinal tract may be involved. Many patients who have had a course of antibiotics, especially the tetracyclines, have prolonged fungal infections of the anus and perianal area. Not only food allergens but highly spiced foods may cause pruritus ani.

Asthma and Nasal Allergy

In many allergic diseases, eczema and urticaria for example, too much attention is often paid to foods. In respiratory allergy the opposite is true—attention is often directed entirely toward inhalants, respiratory irritants, infection, psychic factors, and exercise. In all but the most obvious cases of pure inhalant sensitivity, food allergy should be considered. This is especially true if thickened secretions are present in the nose, throat, bronchi, or middle ears.

Tension-fatigue Syndrome

Although food allergy is a common cause of tension and fatigue, a wide variety of organic and nonorganic influences need to be considered. Few, if any, of these patients tolerate nicotine and many do not tolerate caffeine. Inhalant allergy may also be a factor, and hyposensitization often provides considerable relief.

THE USE OF DRUGS

In dealing with food allergy, our interest in drugs centers almost exclusively on the reactions they may cause rather than on the relief of symptoms they may provide. It is true that such drugs as sympathomimetics, corticosteroids, antihistamines, and theophylline are indicated in temporarily relieving various allergic diseases, but they play no part in specific treatment. Experienced victims of food allergy are aware of this, and when they are careless about eating forbidden foods, they learn that the resultant symptoms will generally subside spontaneously. The only significant exception is a reaction to a food so violent that it requires an injection of epinephrine.

In summary it may be said that the treatment of food allergy depends chiefly on the detection and elimination of the offending foods, the degree of elimination depending on the patient's tolerance. But since food allergy is rarely the patient's only problem, the importance of other allergic and nonallergic causes must not be overlooked. It must also be remembered that the patient requires a palatable and nourishing diet, including, if necessary, vitamin and mineral supplements. The important subject of providing such a diet is the concern of the next chapter.

8 • ALLERGIC COOKERY

In many cases of food allergy, avoidance is no problem. A person allergic to walnut, chocolate, or shrimp, for example, needs no help whatever; he simply avoids the offending foods completely. It is primarily to help patients who are allergic to common foods, such as milk, corn, wheat, and egg, that this chapter is written. When faced with the problem of providing a nourishing and acceptable diet for these patients we naturally turn to foods they *can* eat.

This chapter is organized as a concise encyclopedia of common foods, both those that are important allergens and those that are not. Listed individually are milk, egg, chocolate, grains, and the common meats, vegetables, and fruits. Other headings are *Nuts, Oils, Spices, Starches,* and *Sugars.* An important separate heading is *Soups, Stews, and other mixed dishes.* These foods add variety to the diet of those with multiple food allergy. If a given food is a common allergen, substitutes are recommended. If it is not a common allergen, ways of using it as a substitute for the more common food allergens are described.

ALMOND

Patients who cannot eat peanut or walnut can almost always eat almond. It can be used in any recipe calling for nuts.

APPLE

Next to the citrus fruits, apple is the most common fruit allergen. It is especially likely to cause trouble when eaten raw and unpeeled. Cider (apple juice) and cider vinegar are also common offenders. Many apple-sensitive patients have complete tolerance for cooked apple in such desserts as apple pie and apple sauce. Since distilled vinegar is derived from grain alcohol, it can be used in place of cider vinegar; salads made with wine vinegar are especially delicious.

ARROWROOT

Used in place of corn starch and wheat flour, arrowroot flour is an excellent thickening agent for such foods as soups, gravies, and stews. It may be mixed with a small amount of water and stirred into broth.

This is done at the end of the cooking time when the liquid is just coming to a boil. (It tends to lose its thickening power if overcooked.)

ARTICHOKE

Also known as the globe artichoke (to distinguish it from the Jerusalem artichoke), this hypoallergenic vegetable is a welcome addition to the diet of patients with multiple food allergy. The receptacle and bracts ("leaves") of the flowering head make up the edible part. Canned and frozen artichoke hearts may be used as a cooked vegetable or may be marinated as follows: Combine oil, vinegar, salt, and Italian herb seasoning. (Spice Islands and McCormick Italian herb dressings contain marjoram, thyme, rosemary, savory, oregano, sage, and basil.) Wash and drain the hearts and place in marinade for at least 15 minutes, preferably longer.

Fresh artichoke may be the most delicious of all vegetables. It may be prepared as follows:

> Wash under running water. Cut off stem and about ½ inch of the top and remove the small bottom leaves. Cut off tips of remaining leaves with kitchen shears. Boil in sufficient salted water to half cover, and cook until an outer leaf may easily be plucked (30–40 minutes). To serve, place on a plate with a small cup of lemon butter. One at a time each leaf is plucked and dipped in sauce. The fleshy base of the leaf is placed between the teeth and sheared off when the leaf is pulled away. When all leaves have been discarded, the base is cut in two with a sharp knife, and the spiny center is discarded. The remaining bottom, the most delicious part of the vegetable, is then eaten after being dipped in sauce. (Note to the cook: You may want to wear gloves when preparing artichokes since they tend to stain the fingers an unsightly brown. The stain, however, can be removed with lemon juice.)

ARTICHOKE, JERUSALEM

This vegetable resembles the true artichoke in name only. The edible portion is the tuber. Jerusalem artichoke grows readily in the home garden as a somewhat weedy perennial.

Raw Jerusalem artichokes are crisp and crunchy with a delicate, nutty flavor. They are good sliced in salads or eaten like radishes or carrot sticks. To cook, slice in ¼- to ½-inch slices and boil for about 5 minutes in a small amount of water with salt and 1 or 2 teaspoonsful of lemon juice. Do not overcook as the crispy texture will be lost. Add butter and serve. Jerusalem artichokes add interest to soups and stews and may be stir-fried alone or with other vegetables.

ASPARAGUS

Asparagus may on occasion cross-react with onion, garlic, and other members of the lily family, but this is unusual. It is accordingly an excellent vegetable for most patients with multiple food allergy. When bought in the market it is inclined to be expensive. For this reason, everyone who enjoys gardening should try to make space for an asparagus bed.

To prepare fresh asparagus for cooking, snap off the lower part of the stalk; it will break at the point where it becomes tender. Because grit will cling under the scales, asparagus must be washed thoroughly. At times it is necessary to remove the scales to get rid of the grit. The simplest and best way to cook asparagus is to steam or boil for 5 minutes or until tender. Salt and butter are then added.

AVOCADO

Avocado adds both variety and nourishment to the diet. It may be used in salads and in various dips. A simple method of preparing avocado is to slice the fruit into strips and lay on a salad plate. Squeeze lemon juice or wine vinegar on the strips and add plain or seasoned salt. A sprinkling of Italian herb seasoning may also be used.

BANANA

This popular fruit is a fairly common allergen when eaten raw but rarely, if ever, is allergenic after being cooked. It can be used in breads, cakes, and pies. A tendency for banana to cause indigestion and mouth irritation does not seem to be related to allergy.

BARLEY

Patients allergic to wheat and rice are almost always allergic to barley. In the United States its use is confined mostly to the preparation of malt, beer, and ale. It is used to some extent in soups. An excellent and nutritious substitute is whole buckwheat or buckwheat groats (kasha). (See Buckwheat.)

BEANS

It is unfortunate that the many varieties of beans are such common allergens. For those able to eat these vegetables, however, variety in the diet may be obtained by using a wide selection, such as navy bean, kidney bean, pinto bean, broad bean, soybean, lentil, green pea, split pea, black-eyed pea, crowder pea, garbanzo, and peanut.

BEEF

Most patients with even extensive food allergy are able to eat beef. To add variety to the diet, wider use should be made of the less common and less expensive cuts. As an example of such uses, here are methods of preparing beef tongue and oxtails.

> *Beef tongue:* The best tongues weigh 3 pounds or less. Wash the tongue and place it in a 5-quart pan or dutch oven in about 2 inches of water. Bring to a boil over high heat and then turn burner down to medium or low, using sufficient heat to maintain a gentle boil. Skim off gray foam, and using a paper towel wipe foam from sides of pan. After 1 hour, add a carrot cut into chunks, tops of three ribs of celery (leaves included), and an onion cut into chunks. Continue boiling for 2 hours, adding water as needed. At the end of 3 hours the bones should drop from the meat and the skin should be loose enough to be easily removed. If not, continue boiling a bit longer. Remove the skin and trim the base. Return the meat to the pan and place on the burner. Add ½ cup of the broth and ½ cup of burgundy wine (or similar dry red wine) and allow to cook dry over a medium burner. As the pan begins to sizzle and brown, add a small amount of water or wine, tipping the pan to rinse loose the browned particles. Repeat several times until both meat and pan are nicely browned. Remove meat, place on plate, and slice. Make gravy in the pan. Horseradish sauce may be used to enhance the flavor.
>
> *Oxtails:* Oxtails may be braised in the same manner as tongue and served with vegetables. They make excellent soup. To make soup, use the braised meat, add a quart of water to the pan plus any broth left from the first step. This should make about 2 quarts. Bring to a boil and add 4 sliced carrots, 4 ribs of celery, chopped (with leaves), 1 medium onion, ½ cup buckwheat or barley groats. Allow to boil gently until

vegetables and groats are cooked (12–20 minutes). Add a can of green beans with their juice and ¼ cup sherry. Adjust seasoning, adding pepper if desired. A slightly thickened soup may be made by adding ½ cup of dehydrated potato buds or flakes. Stir in and allow the soup to simmer 5–10 minutes.

BEER

Allergy to beer is common, but the responsible allergen or allergens cannot always be identified. The most likely offenders are corn, yeast, alcohol, and barley malt. People who like a light alcoholic drink may use such wines as burgundy and chablis mixed, if desired, with club soda or ginger ale.

BEET

Both the root and leaves of this plant are excellent vegetables. Easily grown in the home garden, they are especially delicious when fresh. They rarely cause allergic reactions.

BLUEBERRY

Blueberry is a hypoallergenic fruit that deserves more extensive use.

BROCCOLI

Perhaps no vegetable has so increased in popularity in recent years as this member of the hypoallergenic mustard (cabbage) family. It is used as a main vegetable and as an ingredient of mixed meat and vegetable dishes. It is available both fresh and frozen and may be grown in the home garden.

BRUSSELS SPROUTS

This, another member of the mustard family, is available both fresh and frozen.

BUCKWHEAT

Buckwheat is totally unrelated to wheat and is therefore a useful substitute. Although not a common allergen, buckwheat is capable of causing severe reactions.[70,121] The following recipe may be used in preparing buckwheat pancakes and waffles for wheat-sensitive patients: (See also Buckwheat Soup under the heading of Soups, Stews. . . .)

Buckwheat Pancakes (and Waffles)

4 cups lukewarm water
1 packet compressed yeast
buckwheat flour (pure buckwheat; no wheat!)
1 tablespoon brown sugar or molasses
2 tablespoons vegetable oil
1½ teaspoon salt
1½ teaspoon baking soda

Soften yeast in 1 cup water, add sugar, salt, 3 cups water, and enough buckwheat flour to make a thin batter. Cover and let rise overnight. (Be sure to use a large container as the batter *does* rise.) Just before cooking, dissolve the baking soda in 1 tablespoon water and add to batter. Beat thoroughly and fry cakes on a hot griddle. Save leftover batter for starter. Store in refrigerator in container at least twice the size necessary as the batter will rise vigorously. If egg is tolerated, add a beaten egg to batter just before frying cakes. To make waffles, add a bit more buckwheat to make a thicker batter.

CABBAGE

This hypoallergenic and relatively inexpensive vegetable has a wide variety of uses as a salad, main vegetable, and ingredient of mixed dishes. Sauerkraut also has a wide variety of uses.

CARROT

Although raw carrot occasionally causes severe reactions, cooked carrot is hypoallergenic.

CELERY

Like the closely related carrot, celery causes trouble chiefly when eaten raw. As a cooked vegetable it may be used in chow mein, soups, stews, and other mixed dishes.

CHERRY

Whether used fresh, canned, frozen, or as a juice, cherry is a welcome addition to the diet of patients with extensive food allergy. On rare occasions it acts as a potent allergen.

CHEWING GUM

This popular confection contains so many ingredients that it is often impossible to identify offending allergens (see page 69). The most common are artificial rubber, chicle, cinnamon, peppermint, and corn syrup.

CHICKEN

As is true of the meat of other birds and of mammals, fish, and crustaceans, allergy to chicken is inclined to be severe. However, chicken is not a common allergen and, like turkey, is a relatively inexpensive and nourishing food for most allergic patients.

CHIVES

Although related to the common allergens onion and garlic, chives rarely, if ever, cross-react with them. They are easily grown as house plants and add welcome flavor to mixed dishes and salads.

CHOCOLATE

Chocolate and its close relative cola are second only to milk as the most common allergens. The presence of chocolate is so obvious to patients that they need no help in avoiding it. Cola extract is present in drinks that have the word "cola" in their name and in Tab. Chocolate substitutes made with carob bean flour are available, but most people do not find them especially appealing. However, we have found brownies made according to the following recipe* to be delicious. Although the brownies do not have a particularly chocolatelike flavor, children often appreciate such treats.

Carob Brownies

2 sticks butter or margarine
2 cups sugar
4 eggs

---

*Recipe by Mrs. Linda Coulter Lundy.

1½ cups flour
6 tablespoons carob powder*
1 tablespoon vanilla
2 cups chopped nuts

Preheat oven to 350⁰ F; grease and flour a 9-inch by 13-inch pan. Cream butter and sugar in a large mixing bowl. Add eggs one at a time, mixing well after each addition. Sift together flour and carob powder and add gradually to egg mixture. Add vanilla and nuts. Pour into prepared pan and bake about 30 minutes until center is firm. Frost when cool, using the following recipe.

Carob Frosting

3 cups powdered sugar (contains trace of cornstarch)
⅓ cup carob powder
1 scant teaspoon instant coffee powder
1 stick soft butter or margarine
¼ cup evaporated milk or light cream

Sift together sugar, carob powder, and instant coffee powder; set aside. Cream butter until fluffy; add evaporated milk. Gradually add mixed dry ingredients, beating well after each addition. For thinner frosting add more milk.

COFFEE

Coffee is an occasional allergen, especially in allergic headache. In the case of most people who cannot take coffee, the reaction more properly may be termed idiosyncrasy, the common reactions being indigestion, palpitation, tremor, restlessness, and insomnia. Such complaints are not always relieved when decaffeinated coffee is used. Patients who like a hot beverage with a somewhat similar flavor may find Postum an acceptable substitute.

COLLARDS

This relative of cabbage deserves more general use. Many people consider collard greens more delicious than spinach or Swiss chard.

---

*Carob powder is available from health food stores or from El Molino Mills, PO Box 2250, City of Industry, Calif. 91746.

COLORS

The most important sources of artificial food colors are drinks such as Tang, Hawaiian Punch, and Kool Aid. Popsicles and colored gelatin desserts (Jello) are also important. The substitution of natural fruits and juices will make the use of these products unnecessary. They can be used "as is," frozen, or incorporated into uncolored gelatin.

CORN

Corn (maize) is an especially common and potent allergen and one that is easily overlooked. The many ways corn may appear in foods is shown in Table 6-3. Since it is impossible to list all foods that contain corn, especially corn syrup (corn sweetener), the patient must make it his responsibility to read labels carefully. Since labeling is not always accurate, it must be assumed that sweetened foods and baked goods contain corn syrup until proved otherwise.

Patients vary as to the type of corn to which they are allergic. Some cannot take it in any form except pure corn sugar (glucose). Others have no trouble with immature corn, that is to say, corn on the cob and canned (either kernel or cream-style) corn. Corn syrup, for some obscure reason, is the most potent offender; corn oil the least. Some patients can eat popcorn and other whole corn products but not corn syrup.

Since corn syrup is so commonly used and is so potent an allergen, those who prepare foods for corn-sensitive patients need guidance in avoiding it when preparing sweetened foods. For this reason, *none* of the recipes in this chapter contain corn syrup. The following recipes show how candies and spreads may be prepared without its use.

Strawberry Preserves

4 cups fresh strawberries, quartered
5 cups sugar
½ cup water
¼ bottle Certo

Mix first three ingredients in a large pan (8-quart or more) and put on medium burner until a juice forms. Turn heat to high and bring to a full, rolling boil, stirring constantly. Boil 2–3 minutes. Be sure all sugar crystals are off sides of pan. Remove from heat and add Certo, stirring constantly. Pour in-to a large bowl and stir, skimming until all foam is removed

(5–10 minutes). Cover bowl and let stand several hours, stirring every 10–15 minutes until cool. Place in sterilized jars and cover immediately with melted paraffin. Cover with lids, label, and store in a cool, dark place.

Burnt Almond Candy

1½ cups almonds with skins on
1 cup water
1 cup sugar
1 tablespoon butter
¼ teaspoon salt
¼ teaspoon soda

In a heavy skillet or 2-quart sauce pan (cast aluminum *without* Teflon, or a heavy iron pan) combine almonds, salt, sugar, and water. Bring to boil, stirring until sugar melts. Reduce heat to low and simmer until almonds make a popping noise (15–20 minutes). Remove from heat and add butter and soda. Stir until sugar crystallizes (mixture will become dry). Return to heat and cook over low to medium heat until sugar starts to melt and clings to almonds to form a glaze (about 10 minutes). Turn out onto greased cookie sheet and separate almonds with two forks. Allow to cool completely, then store in airtight containers in a cool, dry place. (Note: other nuts, such as large peanuts or filberts, may be used.)

Peanut Brittle

2 cups sugar
1 cup water
2 cups raw peanuts
1 teaspoon salt
⅛ teaspoon cream of tartar
1 tablespoon butter
1½ teaspoons soda (measure onto a saucer and crush lumps.)

Combine sugar, water, salt, cream of tartar, and peanuts in a heavy, deep skillet or 4-quart pan and bring to boil over high heat, stirring until sugar melts. Reduce heat to low and simmer mixture. Place candy thermometer in pan. Remove crystals from sides of pan. Add butter when thermometer reaches 170° F, stirring enough to mix. The mixture will begin to form crystals at about 190° F. At this point turn the heat to medium and stir gently with a folding motion. As the sugar caramelizes, the crystals disappear. For this part you may like to use a wooden spoon. Be sure all crystals are dissolved and none remain on pan or spoon. This must be done quickly as the candy is very hot (about 306° F). Remove from heat and add soda, stirring just enough to blend. When candy foams up, pour onto a large, lightly oiled cookie sheet and spread quickly with spatula. Be careful—this candy is hot!

CRANBERRY

Since cranberry is hypoallergenic, cranberry juice and sauce are useful in planning a diet for many patients. It may be blended with other fruit juices.

CRUSTACEANS

Allergy to shrimp, lobster, crab, and other crustaceans is almost always severe, and cross-reactivity is usually complete. Patients often do not realize that allergy to crustaceans has nothing to do with allergy to fish or to clams, oysters, and other mollusks.

CUCUMBER

As is true of many foods of plant origin, cucumber is more likely to cause indigestion than true allergy. It may be allergenic when eaten raw but not when pickled or cooked.

DATE

Although not a popular fruit in the Western world, date is useful in adding variety and nourishment to what may sometimes be a monotonous diet. Allergy to date is uncommon.

EGG

Avoiding egg as such (boiled, poached, coddled, fried, scrambled) is no problem, but egg in cooking calls for the use of substitutes. This is especially true of such baked goods as cakes and cookies. The following recipes are offered for patients who must be strict in their avoidance of egg:

Eggless Chocolate Cake

1 cup sugar
3 tablespoons butter or margarine
1 cup sifted wheat flour
3 tablespoons cocoa
1 teaspoon baking powder
¼ teaspoon salt
½ cup milk
½ teaspoon vanilla

In a small mixing bowl, cream sugar and shortening and about 1 tablespoon of the milk until light. Add the sifted dry ingredients alternately with milk, ending with dry. Beat for at least two minutes. Pour into greased and floured 9-inch round cake pan. Bake in 350° F oven for 35 minutes or until done. (See also Honey Cake and Pineapple Cookies under Wheat.)

Eggless Mayonnaise

1 teaspoon salt
1 teaspoon paprika
1 teaspoon sugar
1 teaspoon dry mustard
¼ cup evaporated milk
¾ cup vegetable oil (soy, safflower, olive, etc)
2 teaspoons lemon juice or vinegar (apple, distilled, wine)

Chill all liquids and bowl. Mix dry ingredients. Add to milk in small mixer bowl. Beat at high speed while adding 1 table-spoon of oil slowly in a fine stream as for regular mayonnaise. Add lemon juice or vinegar, a small amount at a time, alternately with rest of oil. Beat well after each addition. Store in jar in refrigerator. This mayonnaise has excellent flavor but is not as stable as that made with egg.

ELDERBERRY

This fruit, which grows wild in many parts of the United States, may be used to make jelly and wine. It has a distinct flavor that is relished by many people.

FIG

Like date (an entirely unrelated fruit), fig may be used to add variety to a monotonous diet.

FISH

No fish-sensitive patient is unaware of his problem or needs help in avoiding its source. He may not know, however, that he *may* be able to eat oysters, shrimp, and lobster. And patients unable to eat one type of fish may be able to eat others (see Chapters 4 and 5).

GARBANZO

This legume, also known as chick pea, makes a welcome addition to the diet of patients able to eat the seeds of this family. It may be used as an appetizer with oil, vinegar, and Italian herb dressing.

GOOSEBERRY

Gooseberry is used in pies and tarts. Allergy to gooseberry and its close relative currant has not been reported.

GRAPE

Patients allergic to grape must avoid not only raw grapes but grape juice, grape jellies and jams, raisins, and grape wine. Patients who like wine may want to try wines made from other fruits. In most cases, however, it is the alcohol in wines rather than the fruit itself that causes the patient's symptoms.

HONEY

The allergenicity of honey seems to depend on contaminants from the plant furnishing the bee with nectar. Since most honey in this country is gathered from the pea family, patients allergic to beans, peas, and peanut may be allergic to honey. Honey is useful as a substitute for corn syrup in pancake syrup and candies.

HORSERADISH

If it is eaten in quantity, horseradish is poorly digested, but as it is ordinarily used, it adds piquancy to many meat and vegetable dishes.

KOHLRABI

People who have tried kohlrabi rank it high among the more desirable vegetables. It is especially delicious when eaten raw. When cooked, it has a flavor resembling that of its close relative turnip. It is very easily grown in the home garden.

LAMB

For patients allergic to beef or pork, lamb is a useful and delicious substitute. In general, it may be used in place of any other meat in standard recipes, but most cooks use more garlic and spices in cooking lamb than they do with beef or pork. (Lamb Stew is listed under Soups, Stews. . . .)

LENTILS

Patients who tolerate legumes will find lentil soup a nourishing and tasty dish.

LETTUCE

Patients allergic to lettuce tend to forget that it is not a necessary ingredient of salads. As the leafy part of a salad, cabbage, including Chinese cabbage and savoy cabbage, may be substituted. Other foods that may be used in salads are tomato, green pepper, hot pepper, celery, carrot, radish, cauliflower, spinach, apple, lemon juice, pickled beets, melon, chives, onion, cucumber, watercress, garden cress, parsley, endive, olive, bacon, ham, tuna, and anchovy. These foods, along with seasoned salt and a variety of spices, make possible the preparation of a tremendous variety of salads.

MANGO

This tropical fruit is becoming increasingly popular in this country. It is related to poison ivy, and the skin of the fruit may cause severe dermatitis in patients sensitive to this family of plants.

MARGARINES

Since margarines are made almost exclusively from vegetable oils, allergic reactions may occur in patients allergic to soy, peanut, cottonseed, and corn oils. The patient allergic to one of these oils can usually choose a margarine made from another. Butter contains so little milk that it is virtually nonallergenic, but there are rare exceptions.

MILK

Although cow's milk is by far the most common food allergen, it is usually not an especially potent one. Milk-sensitive patients should not drink it as a beverage and must avoid buttermilk, 2% milk, skim milk, cream, creamed foods, sherbet, ice cream, yogurt, and all types of cheese. Traces of milk in such foods as butter and baked goods may almost always be ignored. As is true of egg allergy, milk allergy may be low grade, the patient being able to take a moderate amount every four or five days. This degree of tolerance has an unfortunate tendency to tempt the patient to become careless in avoidance.

Milk can be replaced in many of its uses by nondairy coffee creamers. When coffee creamers are used on cereals, children usually prefer that they be diluted slightly with water. Parents need to be reminded that coffee creamers have little food value and do not replace milk proteins. Fortunately, milk-sensitive people generally are fond of such high-protein foods as meats, fowl, fish, and eggs.

MUSHROOMS

Although low in nutritional value, mushrooms add welcome variety and interest to the diet.

NUTS

The term nut is applied to a variety of seeds, not all of which are true nuts. Those most likely to act as allergens are peanut (actually a legume, not a nut), walnut, pecan, Brazil nut, hazelnut (filbert), and coconut. Less common offenders are almond, cashew, pistachio, macadamia nut, and pinyon nut.

OATS

Oats have some tendency to cross-react with the other small grains. Sometimes they are the only member of the grass family a patient can eat. At other times they are the only grain a patient cannot eat.

OILS

Although lipids are not supposed to be allergenic, vegetable oils can cause severe reactions. Examples of potent offenders are peanut oil, cottonseed oil, and soy oil. Corn oil tends to cause mild reactions, and olive oil and safflower oil appear to be entirely nonallergenic. (See also Margarines.)

OKRA

This Southern favorite is becoming more popular throughout the country. Recipes for its use are found in standard cookbooks.

ONION

Onion and its close relative garlic are fairly common allergens, especially in allergic headache. Most onion-sensitive patients tolerate small amounts, and onion and garlic salts seem to cause none at all.

PAPAYA

Like mango, papaya is a tropical fruit whose use is increasing. No reports of allergy have appeared.

PARSNIP

Allergy to this relative of carrot and celery has not been reported.

PEA

Green (English) pea is not as likely to cause allergic reactions as are mature legumes. At times, however, it is a severe offender and may even be the only legume the patient needs to avoid. Crowder pea, black-eyed pea, and chick pea (garbanzo) are more closely related allergenically to the common bean (navy, pinto, kidney) than to green peas.

PEACH

Peach and its close relative nectarine may be the most delicious of all fruits. They seldom act as allergens.

PEANUT

Patients allergic to peanut are usually well aware of the fact and make a point of avoiding it in all its forms, including peanut butter. However, they may be unaware of the likelihood of their being allergic to other legumes, especially the closely related soybean. (See also Nuts.)

PEPPERS

Green pepper (also known as sweet or mango pepper) commonly causes indigestion but seldom, if ever, acts as a true allergen. Red pepper, an uncommon offender, may be substituted for the unrelated black pepper, a common offender.

PINEAPPLE

Pineapple is often a source of indigestion and is a fairly common allergen. Pineapple juice can often be substituted for orange juice in cases of citrus fruit allergy.

PLUM

Like its relatives peach, apricot, cherry, and almond, plum is not a common allergen. It is used in the preparation of jellies and jams and is the source of prune and prune juice.

PORK

Patients allergic to pork are usually well aware of the fact. Some patients have more trouble from fresh pork, others from cured pork. For some reason, pork roast may be an especially severe offender. Pork is a constituent of sausages, wieners, frankfurters, Vienna sausages, lunch ham, ham spreads, various cold cuts, bacon, and lard.

POTATO

The Irish, or white, potato is a fairly common allergen with some apparent cross-allergenicity with tomato and eggplant. Since its presence in foods is obvious, patients need little guidance in avoidance. In the case of those who cannot eat potato chips and french fried potatoes, the offending allergen may be the vegetable oil in which they are fried.

PUMPKIN

Pumpkin allergy is rare. Patients who have trouble from pumpkin pie usually prove to be allergic to the cinnamon it contains. Here is a recipe for salted pumpkin seeds.

Heat about 1 inch of vegetable oil in a heavy 10-inch skillet over low heat. Test for proper heat by dropping a pumpkin seed into the oil. It should go to the bottom, sizzle, and rise to the top where it will swell and probably pop. Add ½ cup of pumpkin seeds at one time to the hot oil (use low heat because the seeds burn easily). As soon as all rise to the top, remove with slotted spoon, drain on paper towel, and salt. Pumpkin seeds make good substitutes for popcorn and peanuts.

RABBIT

Domestic rabbit may be used to supplement the diet of patients allergic to other meats.

RHUBARB

Served like a fruit, this tart vegetable can be used as a substitute for strawberry, apple, and orange.

RICE

Most wheat-sensitive patients are also allergic to rice. If not, they stand a good chance of becoming sensitive to it if they use it as a wheat substitute. For this reason, patients who are allergic to wheat should eat rice sparingly, if at all.

RUTABAGA

Properly prepared, rutabaga is a palatable and nutritious root vegetable. Some people consider it delicious.

RYE

Since there is little cross-reactivity between rye and the other grains, it makes a useful wheat substitute. Ry-Krisp and similar Scandinavian rye "crisp breads" are available in most areas. The ordinary rye bread found in markets contains more wheat flour than rye flour. Pure rye bread may sometimes be found in specialty stores. The following recipe may be used to bake it at home.

Rye Batter Bread

2 packages dry yeast
1½ cups warm water

2 tablespoons shortening

2 tablespoons sugar

3–4 cups rye flour (use Martha Gooch brand if it is available)

¼ cup potato flour

2 tablespoons soybean flour

1 tablespoon salt

In a large mixer bowl, dissolve yeast in warm water. Add shortening, sugar, salt, 2 cups of the rye flour, and all of the potato and soybean flours. Blend on low speed. Beat 2 minutes at medium speed. Stir in remaining flour until you have a very thick and sticky batter. It should be thick enough to stand the spoon up in. Cover and let rise in a warm place for about one hour.

Stir down until all of the air is out. Spread into a well-greased 8-inch loaf pan. Cover loosely with plastic wrap and let rise for about 30–45 minutes. Its appearance will be somewhat dimply. Put into a 350° F oven and bake about 40 minutes or until loaf sounds hollow when pan is tapped on bottom. Remove from pan by running a knife around the outside of the loaf, then knocking the pan sharply on the counter. Reverse pan and knock loaf out. Brush top with butter and cool on a rack.

Tips for success with rye bread: Make sure you add enough flour; it should be quite hard to handle. Let rise until it is double the first rising. When rising the second time, it should not rise quite double. After loaf has cooled, wrap well since it has no preservatives and will dry out.

SALADS

(See Lettuce.)

SOUPS, STEWS AND OTHER MEAT-VEGETABLE DISHES

Those who cook for someone with multiple food allergy need to become expert in using a wide variety of meats, vegetables, and spices in the preparation of soups, stews, and similar dishes. This calls for imagination, ingenuity, experimentation, and willingness to depart from rigid adherence to cookbooks. Here are recipes and suggestions that have proved helpful.

Buckwheat Soup

4 cups water
½ cup buckwheat, whole or groats (kasha)
2–3 bouillon cubes
2 tablespoons Worcestershire sauce
¼ teaspoon oregano
¼ teaspoon thyme
2 tablespoon chopped onion
2 ribs celery

Mix all ingredients in large pan and cook over medium heat until buckwheat is done (about 20–30 minutes). Whole buckwheat has more flavor than groats; both are available in Jewish delicatessens and many supermarkets.

Chili Zucchini (no tomato)

1 pound ground chuck
1 can (16 ounces) red beans
1 tablespoon chili powder
2 tablespoons vinegar or lemon juice
½ cup water
2–3 medium-size zucchini squash, sliced

Steam ground beef; add beans, chili powder, vinegar and salt to taste. Simmer for 30 minutes to blend flavors. A small amount of water may need to be added to prevent sticking. Add squash and ½ cup water and toss. Cover and cook until squash is tender crisp (8–10 minutes). Adjust seasonings and serve. Leftover chili may be used. This dish may be prepared in a casserole and baked covered in a 350° F oven until it bubbles, about a half hour.

Lamb Stew (no grains or tomato)

bacon fat
2 lamb shanks
3 carrots, ½-inch slices
3 ribs celery, ½-inch slices
1 onion, sliced

2 medium potatoes, ½-inch slices
1 cup okra, frozen or fresh
1 can green beans, drained (save juice)
½ teaspoon oregano
¼ teaspoon marjoram (or substitute Italian
    seasoning for oregano and marjoram)
1 tablespoon tapioca flour
2 tablespoons grainless mix (Cellu)*

Heat a 5-quart dutch oven slowly. Add enough bacon fat to cover bottom of pan. Place shanks in pan and brown slowly, turning frequently. Add a clove of garlic during browning if desired. When nicely browned, discard garlic, drain fat from pan, and add 2 cups of water and herbs, stirring the brown particles loose from bottom of pan. Bring to boil, cover, and cook over low heat until meat is falling from bone (2–3 hours). Remove shanks from pan and remove meat from bone; cut meat into 1-inch pieces. If pan has cooked dry, pour off fat. If not, skim fat from juices. Add enough water to cook vegetables. Add carrots, celery, onion, and potato and cook 5 minutes; then add okra. When all vegetables are tender, add green beans and meat, and simmer. Blend bean juice with tapioca flour and grainless mix and stir into stew. Adjust seasoning and bring to boil. Simmer the stew for several minutes and serve.

Pepper Steaks

½ pound ground chuck
3-4 green peppers
2½ cups water
¼ teaspoon thyme
1 tablespoon tapioca flour
2 tablespoons soy flour or grainless mix (Cellu)
2 teaspoons soy sauce
pinch, seasoned or plain salt

Steam ground beef (don't brown). Prepare green peppers and cut into fourths or smaller. Place peppers in pan with meat and add 1 cup water. Cover and steam until peppers are

---

*Grainless mix is available from Cellu Foods, 1750 West Van Buren St., Chicago, Ill. 60612.

tender. Add remaining water, salt, and thyme. Mix tapioca and soy flour or grainless mix, then blend in soy sauce and ¼ cup water. Add slowly to boiling meat and peppers. Allow to simmer 2–3 minutes. May be served alone or over mashed potatoes or, if grains are allowed, Chinese noodles, egg noodles, or rice. Can also be prepared from frozen peppers.

Stir-Fried Vegetables

2 carrots
2 ribs celery
1 parsnip
1 green pepper
½ can water chestnuts
1 package frozen snow peas (or 2 cups fresh snow peas)
2–3 tablespoons oil

The vegetables should be either thinly sliced (on diagonal for carrots and parsnips) or cut in matchstick-size pieces. Either a wok or 10-inch skillet may be used. Heat the pan until it is very hot and add the oil. A piece of garlic and a slice or two of fresh ginger root may be tossed in the hot oil; they are discarded before the vegetables are added. Start the vegetables that require the longest cooking first, in this case carrots and celery. Toss to coat with oil and continue to cook over high heat about 1 minute; then add the other vegetables and toss to coat with oil. It may be necessary to add a tablespoon or two of water. Continue to stir and cook over high heat about 3 minutes. Add sauce (recipe follows) and toss until it becomes bubbly. The vegetables should be tender crisp.

Any vegetable can be stir-fried. 1) Try adding tomatoes (if allowed), cut in eighths, toward end of cooking time. Be sure to heat through. 2) Add mushrooms, fresh or canned. 3) Add cabbage, Chinese cabbage, spinach, bean sprouts, zucchini, fresh or frozen French style green beans, turnips, or Jerusalem artichokes. Be sure to cut into small pieces.

Meat—beef, chicken, lamb, or pork—can be stir-fried as well. The meat should be cut into thin strips and cooked a bit longer. Remove from pan and keep warm. Stir-fry vegetables with juices and add meat. Use double the amount of sauce as for vegetables alone.

Sauce for Stir-Fried Vegetables

1 teaspoon arrowroot or tapioca flour
¼ teaspoon ground ginger or grated ginger root
½ teaspoon salt
1 tablespoon soy sauce
2 tablespoons dry sherry
1 tablespoon water

Mix and pour over cooking vegetables. Stir until mixture comes to a boil. Serve immediately.

SOYBEAN

This widely used legume, a close relative of peanut, is a great nuisance to those who are allergic to it. Since soy oil is at present the least expensive of the vegetable oils, it is widely used in salad oils, mayonnaise, shortenings, and margarines. Soy protein is being used more and more in all sorts of products, including baked goods, meat extenders, infant "hypoallergenic" formulas, and breakfast cereals.

SPICES

As is true of nuts, spices may be divided into those that commonly cause trouble and those that do not. The most common offenders are cinnamon, black pepper, and bay leaf. Somewhat less important are the mint spices, including peppermint, thyme, and sage, and the parsley spices, especially cumin and coriander. The least common offenders are red pepper, ginger, allspice, mustard, oregano, and clove.

SPINACH

Neither true spinach nor the unrelated New Zealand spinach is inclined to be allergenic. Both can be grown well in the home garden; New Zealand spinach has a long growing season.

SQUASH

Summer squash and winter squash are delicious, nourishing, and hypoallergenic foods. Severely allergic patients who do not already have a taste for these vegetables should acquire it. Squash is easily grown in the home garden.

STARCHES

Since our common food starch is made from corn, a common allergen, substitutes are needed. Soy flour and the starches of potato, arrowroot, and tapioca may be used in place of cornstarch and, in some instances, wheat flour.

SUGARS

Pure sugars derived from cane, beet, and corn are not allergenic. Allergy to corn syrup, however, is very common. Some patients need to avoid brown sugar, sorghum and cane molasses, and honey. Where their flavor is desired, maple sugar and maple syrup may be used.

SWEET POTATO

People may be divided into those who like sweet potato and those who do not. It is a taste that should be cultivated by patients with multiple food allergy.

SWISS CHARD

This relative of spinach and beet makes excellent greens. It is easily grown in the home garden and has the advantage of growing throughout the entire summer.

TEA

Tea is an occasional allergen, but intolerance is usually caused by its content of caffeine. A number of substitutes, such as Kaffir tea and rose hip tea, are available in specialty stores.

TOMATO

Tomato adds an agreeable sweet-sour taste to countless American and foreign dishes. Although its taste cannot be precisely duplicated, the use of sugar and vinegar adds a similar flavor to such dishes as chili con carne and vegetable soup.

TURNIP

Eaten raw or cooked, this hypoallergenic vegetable adds variety to the diet. It does well in the home garden.

WATER CHESTNUT

Water chestnut lends agreeable crispness to salads, Chinese dishes, soups, and stews.

WHEAT

Wheat allergy is a great burden to its victims and to those who prepare their meals. The following flours can be substituted   for wheat flour in gravies, cream sauces, and other dishes requiring thickening: tapioca, arrowroot, rye, soy, or potato starch. In baking, however, no really satisfactory substitute for wheat flour is available. The following recipes are offered for the preparation of baked goods that do not contain wheat, rice, or barley. (See also Buckwheat and Rye.)

Honey Cake (no egg, milk, corn, or grains except rye)

⅓ cup honey
1 cup water
½ cup sugar
2 cups rye flour, finely milled
½ teaspoon baking soda
2 teaspoons baking powder
1 teaspoon cinnamon
½ teaspoon cloves
½ teaspoon allspice
⅛ teaspoon cardamom

Heat first three ingredients in top of double boiler until bubbly. Add to sifted dry ingredients in large mixer bowl and beat for 8-10 minutes. Pour into greased loaf pan and bake in 350⁰ F oven for 50 minutes. Place a pan of water on lowest rack of oven during baking.

This cake resembles lebkuchen and must be stored in an air-tight tin or other container for 3–4 days before it is eaten. An orange icing is good on the cake, or it is good plain or with a little butter.

Pineapple Cookies (no egg, milk, grains, or corn)

½ cup Cellu grainless mix
¼ cup sugar
¼ cup crushed unsweetened pineapple, drained
¼ cup juice from pineapple

Mix all ingredients in bowl and stir until smooth. Drop by teaspoonfuls onto lightly greased cookie sheet and bake in 350° F oven until browned (about 12 minutes). Makes 12 cookies.

Chocolate Chip Cookies (no milk or grains)

1 cup Jolly Joan potato mix (Cellu)
½ cup brown sugar, packed
1 egg
¼ cup butter
½ teaspoon vanilla
1 cup chocolate bits
¼ cup broken nut meats

Place all ingredients in small mixer bowl and mix thoroughly at medium speed. Stir in by hand chocolate bits and nuts. Drop from teaspoon onto lightly greased cookie sheet and bake at 350° F for 12 minutes. Makes 30 medium-size cookies. (Bits should be eliminated for patients with chocolate allergy.)

9 • FOOD ALLERGY IN INFANCY

Food allergy in the first year of life is in several respects different from food allergy in later life. The following are some of the more important differences:

1. Food allergy is characteristically much more severe in infants than in older children and adults. It is an occasional cause of severe anaphylactic shock.[47,67,76,137] This may result in death.[79,107,209]
2. Because of this potential severity and because food allergy in an infant is usually totally unexpected, it tends to cause extreme anxiety in the family.
3. It is easily confused with the infections so prevalent in the early years. This is true of both respiratory and gastrointestinal infections.
4. Unlike food allergy of later life, the history is often of little help.

MANIFESTATIONS

Gastrointestinal

Colic is the most common manifestation of food allergy in infants. Allergic colic differs from the milder "three-month colic" in being severe, persistent, and prolonged. It may continue for as long as two years.[63,176,184]

Projectile vomiting of the type commonly attributed to pylorospasm is another common manifestation; the usual cause is cow's milk.[41,63] Unlike congenital hypertrophic pyloric stenosis, it tends to begin in the neonatal period and may occur at the first feeding.

Constant or intermittent diarrhea is another common manifestation of infantile gastrointestinal allergy. It usually indicates a severe degree of sensitivity to the offending food. Unless there is a complicating infection, the danger of dehydration is usually not great.[63,67,79]

Constipation is the fourth important gastrointestinal allergy of infants. It is more common in later infancy and often follows earlier diarrhea.[41,73] Anal fissure is a common complication.

Other symptoms of food allergy are abdominal distension and bloody diarrhea. Low-grade, occult gastrointestinal bleeding is an important cause of stubborn "iron-deficiency" anemia.[79,214] Many older milk-sensitive children have a history of severe anemia.[214] Perianal excoriation is almost always present in babies with food allergy; it contributes to the high incidence of anal fissure.

Skin

Infantile eczema (atopic dermatitis) is a common and tedious clinical problem. It tends to start during the first month, involving chiefly the cheeks, forearms, and lower legs. At times it is all but generalized, sparing only the palms of the hands and the soles of the feet. It is to be differentiated from seborrhea, candidiasis, and a variety of less common dermatoses.[73] It may occur in phenylketonuria, Leiner's disease, Hurler's syndrome, Wiscott-Aldrich syndrome, Ritter's disease, and various other congenital disorders.

Although not as common as eczema, urticaria may be a manifestation of food allergy in infancy. It sometimes results from contact with foods, but true, cell-mediated contact dermatitis is unusual.

Respiratory Tract

Except for shock the most severe manifestations of food allergy in infants are those involving the nose, pharynx, middle ear, and lower respiratory tract.

Nasal congestion is especially common, and since infants find it difficult to breathe through the mouth, it is more disabling at this age than in later years. It is especially embarrassing to respiration while the baby is nursing the bottle or breast. When there is noticeable nasal discharge, the cause is almost always a viral infection. However, increased *pharyngeal* mucus is commonly caused by foods, especially cow's milk. It is well to rule out congenital choanal atresia and, in older infants, a foreign body, such as a piece of cotton, paper, or cellophane.

The common bronchial reactions to foods are cough, increased secretions, wheezing, and dyspnea.[41] Such manifestations are likely to be serious and call for prompt and vigorous treatment. They are not only important in themselves but are inclined to make the infant susceptible to lower respiratory infection.

Recurrent croup is a fairly common result of food allergy not only in infants but in children as old as three or four years. It is often impossible to determine if croup is the result of allergy or infection; in case of doubt, infection should always be given first consideration.

Increasing attention is being paid to the role of allergy in secretory otitis media.[118,125,145,220] Milk is by far the most common offender.[41,145,220] This disease is one of the most subtle and easily overlooked and also one of the most important manifestations of food allergy.

Constitutional Manifestations

In addition to anaphylactic shock in infants, food allergy causes minor constitutional symptoms such as excessive sweating and salivation, pallor, irritability, and listlessness (tension-fatigue syndrome).[175]

The many manifestations of food allergy in infancy are summarized in Table 9-1. All of these are well documented in the allergic and pediatric literature. The reader will note that many can be caused by other causes than allergy. Especially important are the many gastrointestinal disorders caused by intolerance to carbohydrates, proteins, and lipids. They have been given thorough discussion by Herman and Hagler.[92]

Table 9-1
Manifestations That May Be Caused
by Food Allergy in Infancy

Gastrointestinal
  Colic
  Diarrhea
  Constipation
  Distension
  Bloody stools
  Vomiting
  Proctitis

Skin
  Eczema
  Urticaria
  Vulva irritation
  Perianal excoriation

Respiratory
  Nasal congestion
  Asthma
  Cough
  Secretory otitis media
  Croup

Constitutional
  Shock
  Pallor
  Excessive sweating
  Salivation
  Tension/fatigue

Hematologic
  Hypochromic anemia

MANAGEMENT

Successful management of allergy in infancy depends almost entirely on clinical procedures, that is history and physical examination.[41,67] The physical examination helps determine whether the problem is due to allergy. The history serves the same purpose but also provides leads as to causes. Inquiry as to clinical manifestations may be based on Table 9-1.

Whatever the chief complaint may be, it is the physician's responsibility not only to take care of the manifestations that concern the parents but any others that may be of allergic origin. For example, it is not unusual for a child with eczema to have dyspnea, increased bronchial secretions, and wheezing. These indicate the early stages of asthma, a more important disease than eczema, which is often transient. Another example is the frequent coexistence of severe colic and nasal congestion. The colic will subside in time, but nasal allergy tends to become chronic and to be complicated by middle ear disease.

Inquiry as to causes is directed toward every food the infant has been given; mothers, fortunately, are remarkably dependable in this area. Although the history and elimination diet are the basis of detection of causes, skin testing should always be done.[67,81,93] Despite its limitations (which the parents should be aware of) it can be helpful, often more so than it is in adults. The commonly heard comment, "Babies are too young to be tested," is fallacious.

The following eight allergens may be all that need to be tested. Scratch tests are best for this purpose.

Milk	Egg	Pork	Beef
Peanut	Soybean	Cattle hair	Mold mix

Cattle hair is included because it often suggests milk allergy.[143] The mold inhalant mix is included because mold allergy is not uncommon during the first year of life. Peanut is included because it is a potent allergen that the infant may encounter at an early age in the form of peanut butter.

Such other diagnostic methods as milk precipitin study, total IgE measurement, and RAST are not indicated. Checking precipitin bands, once thought helpful in identifying milk allergy, has been shown to be without value.[68,79,171] Total IgE and RAST not only add little information but are needlessly expensive and invasive.

Since diarrhea caused by food allergy may cause the type of flattening of villi seen in celiac disease, jejunal biopsy has been recommended. Because it is a difficult and invasive test and one not likely to help in the management of these cases, it is contraindicated.[93,188]

After the history, physical examination, differential diagnosis, and skin testing have been checked, I set up the following program.

1. *The formula*—In most cases soy formulas, casein hydrolysates, and, perhaps, goat's milk have already been tried. Fortunately, almost all infants can tolerate at least one kind of meat, so meats are used as the basis of the formula.[73] The mother is instructed in the preparation of the following formula, using a different meat each time. (Since beef is likely to cross-react with cow's milk, it is not used.[73,79])

Home-Made Meat-Base Infant Formula

Boiled water	3 cups (750 ml)
Strained chicken, pork, lamb, rotated	5 oz (150 ml)
Cane or beet sugar	6 tablespoons (90 ml)
Pure cottonseed, safflower, olive, or sunflower oil	4 teaspoons (20 ml)
Tapioca or potato starch (flour)	1 tablespoon (15 ml)
Dicalcium phosphate tablet, crushed	500 mg
Iodized table salt	⅛ teaspoon (500 mg)
Potassium chloride	¼ teaspoon (500 mg)

Instructions
1. Measure ingredients into a bowl and mix with a hand mixer or blender at high speed.
2. Pour desired quantity into scalded bottles; cap.
3. Shake well; refrigerate.
4. Shake bottle and warm to body temperature before feedings. It may be necessary to make cross-cuts in nipples.

Notes
This formula is based on the research of the Gerber Company and made available by them. Approximately 1½ jars of Gerber meats make up the above 5 oz. Dicalcium phosphate must not contain vitamin D. Five hundred-milligram tablets of the pure product are available from Eli Lilly Company. Potassium chloride is available as Featherweight "K" Salt Substitute, Adolf's salt substitute, and No Salt. If soaked one hour before the formula is made, Minute Tapioca may be used as the starch source.

2. Foods known to have caused trouble are withheld and also the following: cereals (wheat, oats, rice, barley), green beans, peas, soy products, orange juice, tomato, and egg.

3. Depending on what the mother has learned about foods that will need to be avoided, a rotation is set up as follows:

First day	Second day	Third day
carrot	sweet potato	squash or beet
pear	plum or peach	banana

If the infant's hunger is not satisfied, he can be given tapioca cooked with sugar and water. It is best to limit formula feedings to five or six ounces. Amounts in excess of this may lead to persistent regurgitation.

4. In ten days or so, rice, oats, and barley cereals are added in rotation. They may be sweetened with sugar.

5. In another ten days, infants over seven or eight months of age may be tried on apple sauce, white potato (dehydrated potatoes may be used), green beans, peas, apricot, and diluted apple, grape, and pineapple juices. If she likes, the mother may feed home-strained asparagus, cauliflower, broccoli, turnip, and other cooked vegetables. Since the above formula and all milk substitutes are always under some suspicion of being incomplete feedings, as wide a variety as possible of meats, vegetables, cereals, and fruits should be used. A vitamin supplement is given as indicated and as tolerated.

If the infant has diarrhea, it can be assumed that there is temporary disaccharidase deficiency.[67,93] For this reason it may be necessary to withhold cane and beet sugar.

6. To challenge or not to challenge. To anyone intent on proving beyond doubt that an infant reacts to a food, three deliberate challenges have been recommended.[76] In a study of 26 infants with a history of severe milk allergy, Ford and Fergusson found this unworkable. In 21 cases the reactions were so severe that no attempt was made to continue testing.[67] We should no more think of challenging an infant with a food that history shows to have caused a severe reaction than we would think of doing so in any patient who has had a severe reaction following penicillin or aspirin.

FOLLOW-UP

After the infant's dietary restrictions are stabilized, the material in the preceding chapter may be used to give him an appetizing and nutritious diet. The question arises as to whether some of these sensitivities may be outgrown. It is a good rule that those that are unusually severe are almost always permanent. This is especially true of allergy to such animal products as milk, egg, and fish, and of such seed allergens as peanut and soybean. Whenever there is doubt, cautious challenge is justified, beginning with minute amounts of the involved food.

In closing this chapter and this book, let me make one point as strongly as I can: When a patient of any age comes in because of such complaints as headache, nasal congestion, asthma, and gastrointestinal disorders, an infancy history of milk allergy always places milk under the strongest possible suspicion. It is questionable if definite and severe milk allergy is ever outgrown. And it is at all ages by far the most common food allergen.

REFERENCES

1. Allan JW: Case of idiosyncrasy. *Br Med J* 1875;1:98.
2. Allen DH, Baker GJ: Chinese restaurant asthma. *N Engl J Med* 1981;305:1154–1155.
3. Alvarez WC: Food sensitivity and conditions that may be confused with it. *Med Clin North Am* 1929;12:1589–1602 (May).
4. American Academy of Allergy: position statements—controversial techniques. *J Allergy Clin Immunol* 1981;67:333–338.
5. Analytical Records: Kola champagne: non-alcoholic tonic and stimulant. *Lancet* 1890;2:724.
6. Anderson JM: Letter. *Lancet* 1973;1:314.
7. Appel SJ, Szanton VL, Rapaport HJ: Survey of allergy in a pediatric population. *Penn Med J* 1961;64:621.
8. Arbeiter HI: How prevalent is allergy among United States school children?—a survey of findings in the Munster (Indiana) school system. *Clin Pediatr* 1967;6:140.
9. Baer H: Rat mast cell degranulation test. *JAMA* 1974;227:1449.
10. Baer H: In vitro methods in allergy. *Med Clin North Am* 1974;58:85–90.
11. Baer HL: A dermatitis due to aniline dye in a food product. *JAMA* 1934;103:10–11.
12. Baldo BA, Turner KJ: The radioallergosorbent test (RAST). *Med J Austral* 1975;2:871–874.
13. Bazaral M, Orgel HA, Hamburger RN: IgE levels in normal infants and mothers and an inheritance hypothesis. *J Immunol* 1971;107:794.
14. Bell EA: *Toxicants Occurring Naturally in Foods.* Committee on Food Protection, Food and Nutritional Board, National Research Council, National Academy of Sciences. Washington, DC, 1973, ed 2.
15. Benarde MA: *The Chemicals We Eat.* New York, American Heritage Press, 1971.
16. Bender AE: Health foods. *Proc Nutr Soc* 1979;38:163–171.
17. Bendersky G, Lupas JA: Anaphylactoid reaction to ingestion of orange. *JAMA* 1960;173:255–256.
18. Black WC: Flax hypersensitiveness. *JAMA* 1930;94:1064–1065.
19. Blue JA: Facts, frills, fallacies and phobias of food allergy. *South Med J* 1968;61:979–983.
20. Boffey PM: Color additives: botched experiment leads to banning of red dye No. 2. *Science* 1976;191:450–451.
21. Bradley SG, Klika LJ: A fatal poisoning from the Oregon rough-skinned newt *(Taricha granulosa)*. *JAMA* 1981;246:247.
22. Brazeau P in Goodman LS, Gilman A (eds): *The Pharmocological Basis of Therapeutics.* New York, Macmillan, 1965, ed 3, p 879.
23. Brown EA: Sensitivity to grape and grape products, including wine. *Ann Allergy* 1953;11:590.
24. Brown J: How could he do this to me? *Good Housekeeping* 1980;190:36–42 (Feb.).
25. Brues CT: *Insects, Food, and Ecology.* New York, Dover Publications, 1972, p 399.

26. Bulkley LD: Asthma as related to diseases of the skin. *Br Med J* 1885;2: 954–956.
27. Castelain PY: Allergy to color additives. *Médecine et Nutrition* 1977;13(2): 112–113.
28. Chayka JS Jr: Personal communication, 1981.
29. Chen JYP: Chinese health foods and herb tonics. *Am J Chinese Med* 1973; 1:225–247.
30. Chin M: Personal communication, 1981.
31. Clark TW: Spasmodic asthma following use of linseed-meal poultice. *Br Med J* 1872;2:257.
32. Coca AF: *Familial Nonreaginic Food Allergy.* Springfield, IL, Charles C Thomas, 1943, p 96.
33. Cooke RA, Vandeveer A Jr: Human sensitization. *J Immunol* 1916;1:201.
34. Cooke RA: Gastrointestinal allergy. *Bull NY Acad Med* 1933;9:15.
35. Coon JM: Food toxicology. *Modern Medicine,* Nov 30, 1970, pp 103–107.
36. Crook WG in Speer F (ed): *The Allergic Child.* New York, Harper & Row, 1963, p 332.
37. Danis PG: Albuminuria associated with other manifestations of allergy in children. *Urol Cutan Rev* 1941;45:126–128.
38. Darby WJ: Food additives. *J Florida MA* 1979;66:471–475.
39. Davies RJ, Wells ID: Influenza virus vaccine and egg allergy. *Proc Roy Soc Med* 1975;68:218.
40. Davison HM: Allergy of the nervous system. *Q Rev Allerg Appl Immunol* 1952;5:157–188.
41. Deamer WC, Gerrard JW, Speer F: Cow's milk allergy: a critical review. *J Family Pract* 1979;9:223–232.
42. Delaney JC: Response of patients with asthma and aspirin idiosyncrasy to tartrazine (a dye commonly used in the food and drug industries). *Practitioner* 1976;217:285–287.
43. Dennis DT: Jake walk in Vietnam (letter). *Ann Intern Med* 1977;86:665–666.
44. Deraney MF: A periodic syndrome due to milk hypersensitivity. *Ann Allergy* 1967;25:332–336.
45. Derbes VJ: The fixed eruption. *JAMA* 1964;190:765–766.
46. Deschamps E: Uncommon form of idiosyncrasy contra asparagus. *JAMA* 1898;31:128–129.
47. Despres P, Plainfosse B, Papiernic, et al: Les intolerances digestives aux proteines du lait de vache ches l'enfant. *Ann Pediatr* 1971;18:477–478.
48. Deutsch R: Where you should be shopping for your family. *Today's Health,* April, 1972, pp 16–19.
49. Dick R: The treatment of dyspepsia. *Lancet* 1850;2:445–446.
50. Dickinson L, Reichert IL, Ho RCS: Lead poisoning in a family due to cocktail glasses. *Am J Med* 1972;52:391–394.
51. Diefenbach WCL: Don't overlook food poisoning. *Consultant* 1976;16: 207 (Sept).
52. Diver DR: Spasmodic asthma following use of linseed-meal poultice. *Br Med J* 1872;2:257.
53. Dockhorn RJ: Histamine release from the leukocytes of food-allergic individuals using whole food extract antigens. *Ann Allergy* 1969;27:409.

54. Duke WW: Food allergy as a cause of abdominal pain. *Arch Intern Med* 1921;28:151-165.
55. Editorial: Pesticides and preventive medicine. *Br Med J* 1970;4:189.
56. Editorial: Food adulteration. *JAMA* 1887;8:684.
57. Edwards AM, Helming O: A case of severe allergy to pea. *J Allerg* 1941-1942;13:420-422.
58. Eyermann CH: Allergic purpura. *South Med J* 1936;28:341-345.
59. Fassett DW: *Toxicants Occurring Naturally in Foods.* Committee on Food Protection, Food and Nutritional Board, National Research Council, National Academy of Sciences, Washington, DC, 1973, ed 2, p 352.
60. Feinberg SM, Aries PL: Asthma from food odors. *JAMA* 1932;98:2281.
61. Fergus W: Idiosyncrasies. *Lancet* 1869;2:563.
62. Fine AJ: Hypersensitivity reaction to kiwi fruit (Chinese gooseberry, *Actinidia chinensis*). *J Allergy Clin Immunol* 1981;68:235-237.
63. Fischer L: Milk idiosyncrasies in children. *JAMA* 1902;39:247-248.
64. Fisherman EW, Cohen G: Chemical intolerance to butylated hydroxyanisole (BHA) and butylated hydroxytoluene (BHT) and vascular response as an indicator and monitor of drug intolerance. *Ann Allergy* 1973;31:126-133.
65. Fletcher DC: Safety of tenderized meat. *JAMA* 1976;236:970.
66. *Food Additives.* Manufacturing Chemists Association, 1974, p 17.
67. Ford RPK, Fergusson DM: Egg and cows' milk allergy in children. *Arch Dis Child* 1980;55:608-610.
68. Freier S: Paediatric gastrointestinal allergy. *Clin Allergy* 1973;3(Suppl):587-618.
69. Friend WG: The cause and treatment of idiopathic pruritis ani. *Dis Col & Rect* 1977;20:40-42.
70. Frost LC: A case of intense food anaphylaxis. *Med Record* 1915;88:483.
71. Galant SP, Bullock J, Frick OL: An immunological approach to the diagnosis of food sensitivity. *Clin Allerg* 1973;3:363-372.
72. Gerrard JW, Ko CG, Vickers P, et al: The familial incidence of allergic diseases. *Ann Allergy* 1976;36:10-15.
73. Glaser J: *Allergy in Childhood.* Springfield, IL, Charles C Thomas, 1956, p 460.
74. Golbert TM, Patterson R, Pruzansky JJ: Systemic allergic reactions to ingested antigens. *J Allergy* 1969;44:96-107.
75. Golbert TM: A review of controversial diagnostic and therapeutic techniques employed in allergy. *J Allerg Clin Immunol* 1975;56:170-190.
76. Goldman AS, Anderson DW, Sellers WA, et al: Milk allergy. *Pediatrics* 1963;32:425-443.
77. Gould GM, Pyle WL: *Anomalies and Curiosities of Medicine.* Philadelphia, WB Saunders, 1896. Reprinted by Julian Press, 1956, pp 490-493. *Virginia Med Month* 1959;86:586-590.
78. Green RC Jr: Nutmeg poisoning. *Virginia Med Month* 1959;86:586-590.
79. Gryboski JD: Gastrointestinal milk allergy in infants. *Pediatrics* 1967;40:354-362.
80. Hall RL: *Toxicants Occurring Naturally in Foods.* Committee on Food Protection, Food and Nutritional Board, National Research Council, National Academy of Sciences, Washington, DC, 1973, ed 2.
81. Halpern SR, Sellers WA, Johnson RB, et al: Development of childhood

allergy in infants fed breast, soy, or cow milk. *J Allergy Clin Immunol* 1973;51:139–151.

82. Hampton SF: Henoch's purpura based on food allergy. *J Allergy* 1940–1941;12:579–591.
83. Hardin JW, Arena JM: *Human Poisoning from Native and Cultivated Plants.* Durham, NC, Duke University Press, 1969, p 29.
84. Harler CR: *Tea Manufacture.* London, Oxford University Press, 1963, pp 107–114.
85. Hartman AF Sr, Hartman AF Jr, Purkerson, et al: Tremetol poisoning—not yet extinct. *JAMA* 1963;185:706.
86. Hayes CH, Hegsted DM: Toxicity of the vitamins, in *Toxicants Occurring Naturally in Foods.* Committee on Food Protection, Food and Nutritional Board, National Research Council, National Academy of Sciences, Washington, DC, 1973, ed 2.
87. Hedrick UP: *Sturtevant's Edible Plants of the World.* New York, Dover Publications, 1972, pp 96 and 569.
88. Heiner DC: Food allergy; cytotoxic diagnostic technique not proven. *JAMA* 1972;220:1624.
89. Heiner DC: Rat degranulation test. *JAMA* 1974;227:1449.
90. Herbert V: Facts and fictions about megavitamin therapy. *J Florida MA* 1979;66:475–481.
91. Herbert V: The vitamin craze. *Arch Int Med* 1980;140:173–176.
92. Herman RH, Hagler L: Food intolerance in humans. *Western J Med* 1979; 130:95–116.
93. Hill DJ, Davidson GP, Cameron DJS, et al: The spectrum of cow's milk allergy in childhood. *Acta Paediatr Scand* 1979;68:847–852.
94. Hoobler BE: Some early symptoms suggesting protein sensitization in infancy. *Am J Dis Child* 1916;12:129.
95. Hopkins HR: Idiosyncrasy. *Trans Med Soc State New York* 1888;72:78.
96. Horesh AJ: Allergy to food odors. *J Allergy* 1942–1943;14:335–339.
97. Horesh AJ: Buckwheat allergy. *Ann Allergy* 1962;30:685.
98. Ishazaka K, Ishizaka T, Hornbrook M: Physiochemical properties of reaginic antibody. *J Immunol* 1966;99:1187.
99. Jimenez B: A survey of sensitization in students of the University of Michigan. *J Michigan Med Soc* 1934;33:310.
100. Johnstone IL: Apple allergy. *Br Med J* 1972;4:613.
101. Jones BB: Relation of food allergy to nutrition, disease, and behavior in children. *Virginia Med Month* 1949;76:118–120.
102. Jones LW (ed): *A Treasury of Spices.* Baltimore, American Spice Trade Association, 1956, pp 95–129.
103. Juhlin L, Michaelsson G, Zetterstrom O: Urticaria and asthma induced by food-and-drug additives in patients with aspirin hypersensitivity. *J Allergy Clin Immunol* 1972;50:92–98.
104. Jukes TH: How safe is our food supply? *Arch Intern Med* 1978;138: 772–774.
105. Kaplan I: The elusive link in incurable bronchial asthma—food allergy. *South African Med J* 1967;42:1123–1127.
106. Keller E: Chewing gum—a big industry. *Chemistry* 1969;42:16–18.
107. Kelvin CB, Schless RA: Food allergy: death in a six-day-old infant. *J Pediatr* 1948;33:457–461.

108. Kenney RA, Tidball CS: Human susceptibility to oral monosodium L - glutamate. *Am J Clin Nutr* 1972;25:140-146.
109. Kingsbury: Asthma produced by a linseed poultice. *Br Med J* 1885;1:278.
110. Klaw S: Pursuing health in the promised land. *Horizon* 1976;18:24-28.
111. Kleinman AI: Allergy to chicle. *JAMA* 1935;104:455-456.
112. Knox GM: How healthy are health foods? *Better Homes & Gardens* 1972; 50:30-32 (Jan).
113. Kochen J: Sulfur dioxide, a respiratory tract irritant, even if ingested (letter). *Pediatrics* 1974;52:145-146.
114. Koster M, David GK: Reversible severe hypertension due to licorice ingestion. *N Engl J Med* 1968;278:1381-1382.
115. Lapedes DN (ed): *The Spice Cookbook.* New York, David White, 1964.
116. Larm P: Personal communication from Hawaii, 1981.
117. LaRoche G, Richet C Fils: *Alimentary Anaphylaxis.* Translated by Rowe MP, Rowe AH: Berkeley, University of California Press, 1930.
118. Lecks HI: Allergic aspects of serous otitis media. *New York State J Med* 1961;61:2737.
119. Leonard GS: Behavioral manifestations of allergic children. *Ann Allergy* 1966;24:248-249.
120. Lieberman P, Crawford L, Bjelland J, et al: Controlled study of cytotoxic food test. *JAMA* 1975;231:728-740.
121. Lintz W: Gastro-intestinal allergy. *NY State J Med* 1934;34:282-289.
122. Lippe B, Hense L, Mendoza G, et al: Chronic vitamin A intoxication. *Am J Dis Child* 1981;135:634-636.
123. Lockey SD: Allergic reactions due to FD&C yellow No. 5, tartrazine. *Ann Allergy* 1959;17:718.
124. London AH Jr: The composition of an average pediatric practice. *J Pediatr* 1937;10:762.
125. McGovern JP, Haywood TJ, Fernandez AA: Allergy and secretory otitis media. *JAMA* 1967;200:124.
126. Mackie TT: Food allergy in ulcerative colitis. *J Am Dietet Assoc* 1938; 14:177-182.
127. Mahoney CP, Margolis T, Knauss TA, et al: Chronic vitamin A intoxication in infants fed chicken liver. *Pediatrics* 1980;65:893-896.
128. Man-Kwok RH: Chinese restaurant syndrome. *N Engl J Med* 1968;278: 796.
129. Margarine. *Consumer Reports 1976 Buying Guide.* pp 61-67.
130. Matsumura R, Kiroume R, Fukushima I: Significance of food allergy in the etiology of orthostatic albuminuria. *J Asthma Res* 1966;3:325.
131. Méndez JD, del Carril M, Lenci PR: Anafilaxia digestiva por yerba mate. *Revista Asoc Med Argentina* 1933;47:106-108.
132. Meyer LH: *Food Chemistry.* New York, Rheinhold Pub Co, 1960, pp 276-277.
133. Miller JA: *Toxicants Occurring Naturally in Foods.* Committee on Food Protection, Food and Nutritional Board, National Research Council, National Academy of Sciences, Washington, DC, 1973, ed 2, p 539.
134. Miller SA: Additives in our food supply. *Ann New York Acad Sci* 1977; 300:397-405.
135. Morgan JP, Tulloss TC: The jake walk blues. *Ann Intern Med* 1976;85: 804-808.

210

136. Morse RA: Honey. *Natural History.* 1969;78:58.
137. Mortimer EZ: Anaphylaxis following ingestion of soybean. *J Pediatr* 1961;58:90–92.
138. Murray JJ: Milk and peculiar behavior (letter). *Pediatrics* 1979;64:699.
139. Natelson EA, Fred HL: Lead poisoning from cocktail glasses. *JAMA* 1976;236:2527.
140. Nogaller AM, Gorbunov IV: Food allergy in chronic diseases of the digestive tract. *Acta Allergol* 1972;27:145–158.
141. Nunn TW: Idiosyncrasies. *Br Med J* June 11, 1859. Quoted in *Am J Med Sc* 1859;38:547–548.
142. Osler W: The visceral lesions of purpura and allied conditions. *Br Med J* 1914;1:517.
143. Osvath P, Muranyi L, Endre L, et al: Investigation of reactivity of cow hair and milk antigen in bronchial provocation. *Acta Allergol* 1972;27:355–363.
144. Patwardhan VN, White JW Jr: *Toxicants Occurring Naturally in Foods.* Committee on Food Protection, Food and Nutritional Board, National Research Council, National Academy of Sciences, Washington, DC, 1973, ed 2.
145. Phillips BL: Otitis media, milk allergy, and folk medicine (letter). *Pediatrics* 1972;50:346.
146. Pipes DM: The incidence of major and minor allergy in the deep South. *South Med J* 1937;30:1012.
147. Pomeranz Y, Robbins GS: Amino acid composition of buckwheat. *Agr Food Chem* 1972;20:270–274.
148. Powell NB, Powell ER: Vesical allergy in females. *South Med J* 1954;47:841–848.
149. Public Health Laboratory Service (Britain): Unusual outbreak of food poisoning. *Brit Med J* 1976;2:1268.
150. Pugh SM, Rhodes J, Mayberry JF, et al: Atopic disease in ulcerative colitis and Crohn's disease. *Clin Allergy* 1979;9:221–223.
151. Radke D: *Cheese Making in the Home.* Garden City, NY, Doubleday & Co, 1974.
152. Raymond JH: An idioscyncrasy. *JAMA* 1893;21:935–936.
153. Rinkel HJ: Food allergy; function and clinical application of the rotary diversified diet. *J Pediatr* 1948;32:266.
154. Roberts HJ: Perspective on vitamin E as therapy. *JAMA* 1981;246:129–131.
155. Roe FJC: Potential carcinogenic hazards of foodstuffs. *Proc Roy Soc Med* 1973;66:23–25.
156. Roods HA: Letter. *Lancet* 1841;2:717–718.
157. Rowe AH: *Elimination Diets and the Patient's Allergies.* Philadelphia, Lea & Febiger, 1944.
158. Rowe AH: Fever due to food allergy. *Ann Allergy* 1948;6:252.
159. Rubin JM, Shapiro J, Muehlbauer P, et al: Shock reaction following ingestion of mango. *JAMA* 1965;193:397–398.
160. Saarinen UM, Kajosaari M: Does dietary elimination in infancy prevent or only postpone a food allergy? *Lancet* 1980;1:166–167.
161. Schantz EL: *Toxicants Occurring Naturally in Foods.* Committee on Food Protection, Food and Nutritional Board, National Research Council,

National Academy of Sciences, Washington, DC, 1973, ed 2.
162. Schorer EH: Idiosyncrasy to common foods. *J Missouri Med Soc* Dec, 1912, p 1.
163. Schuyler WJ: Discussion on food idiosyncrasies. *New York State J Med* 1917;17:424.
164. Sethi JP, Kasliwal RM, Gupta MM, et al: Significance of food allergens in Indian diet. *J Assoc Physicians India* 1964;12:623–634.
165. Settipane GA, Pudipakkam RK: Aspirin intolerance III. Subtypes, familial occurrence, and cross-reactivity with tartrazine. *J Allergy Clin Immunol* 1975;56:215–221.
166. Shannon WR: Neuropathic manifestations in infants and children as a result of anaphylactic reactions to foods contained in their dietary. *Am J Dis Child* 1922;24:89.
167. Shaywitz BA, Siegel NJ, Pearson HA: Megavitamins for minimal brain dysfunction. *JAMA* 1977;238:1749–1750.
168. Simon AL, Howe R: *Dictionary of Gastronomy.* New York, McGraw-Hill, 1970.
169. Smith HJ: Buckwheat poisoning. *Arch Intern Med* 1909;3:350.
170. Solari MA: Allergia alimentaria. *Rev Med Córdoba* 1954;43:35–42.
171. Soothill JF, in Freier S (ed): Paediatric gastrointestinal allergy. *Clin Allergy* 1973;3(Suppl):616.
172. South MA: The so-called salicylate-free diet: part II. *Cutis* 1976;18:332–333.
173. Speer F: Allergy to methyl salicylate. *Ann Allergy* 1979;43:36–37.
174. Speer F: *The Management of Childhood Asthma.* Springfield, IL, Charles C Thomas, 1951.
175. Speer F: The allergic tension-fatigue syndrome. *Ped Clin N Am* 1954;1:1029–1037.
176. Speer F: Colic and allergy. *Arch Pediatr* 1958;75:271–278.
177. Speer F (ed): *The Allergic Child.* New York, Harper & Row, 1963.
178. Speer F: Allergy and migraine: a clinical study. *Headache* 1971;11:63–67.
179. Speer F, Dockhorn RJ (eds): *Allergy and Immunology in Children.* Springfield, IL, Charles C Thomas, 1973.
180. Speer F: Aspirin allergy: a clinical study. *South Med J* 1975;68:314–318.
181. Speer F: The Bela Schick lecture: The many facets of migraine. *Ann Allergy* 1975;34:273–285.
182. Speer F: Multiple food allergy. *Ann Allergy* 1975;34:71–76.
183. Speer F, Denison TR, Baptist JE: Aspirin allergy. *Ann Allergy* 1981;46:123–126.
184. Stafford HE, Watson RG, Jacobus LR: Abdominal allergy in infancy. *California West Med* 1931;34:168–172.
185. Startin J: Idiosyncrasy to food. *Lancet* 1883;1:348.
186. Stevenson DD, Simon RA: Sensitivity to ingestion of metabisulfites in asthmatic subjects. *J Allergy Clin Immunol* 1981;68:26–32.
187. Strem EL, Stoesser AV: Does honey in infant feeding cause allergy? *Ann Allergy* 1958;16:375–379.
188. Sumithran E, Iyngkoran N: Is jejunal biopsy really necessary in cow's milk protein intolerance? *Lancet* 1977;2:1122–1123.
189. Sure B: Nutritive value of proteins in buckwheat and their role as supplements to proteins in cereal grains. *J Agr Food Chem* 1954;3:793–795.

190. Talbot F: Food idiosyncrasies in practice. *Med Record* 1917;91:875.
191. Thomas JW, Wofford CP: Gastrointestinal allergy—a review of 134 cases. *Am J Digest Dis* 1941;8:311–313.
192. Thornburg WW: Salicylates in canned foods. Study by Del Monte Corporation Research Center, Walnut Creek, CA. Made available 1981.
193. Tolber SG: Food problems. *Cutis* 1981;28:360–367.
194. Torsney PJ: Hypersensitivity to sesame seed. *J Allergy* 1964;35:514–519.
195. Trager J: *The Food Book.* New York, Grossman Publishers, 1970, p 225.
196. Truelove SC: Ulcerative colitis provoked by milk. *Br Med J* 1961;1:154–160.
197. Tuft L, Blumstein GI: Studies in food allergy. *J Allergy* 1946;17:329–339.
198. Tuft L, Girsh LS: Buccal mucosal tests in patients with canker sores (aphthous stomatitis). *J Allergy* 1958;29:502–510.
199. Turnbull JA: The tired, weak, exhausted patient. *Am J Digest Dis* 1943; 87:218–224.
200. Underwood EJ, in *Toxicants Occurring Naturally in Foods.* Committee on Food Production, Food and Nutritional Board, National Research Council, National Academy of Sciences, Washington, DC, 1973, p 159.
201. Unger L: *Bronchial Asthma.* Springfield, IL, Charles C Thomas, 1945, p 159.
202. Unger L, Harris MC: *Stepping Stones in Allergy.* Minneapolis, Craftsman Press, 1975.
203. Van Veen AG, in *Toxicants Occurring Naturally in Foods.* Committee on Food Protection, Food and Nutritional Board, National Research Council National Academy of Sciences, Washington, DC, 1973, ed 2, pp 464–465.
204. Vaughan WT: Minor allergy: Its distribution, clinical aspects, and significance. *J Allergy* 1934;5:184.
205. Vedanthan PK, Menon MM, Bell TD, et al: Aspirin and tartrazine oral challenge: incidence of adverse response in chronic childhood asthma. *J Allergy Clin Immunol* 1977;60:8–13.
206. Weber RW, Hoffman M, Raine DA Jr, et al: Incidence of bronchoconstriction due to aspirin, azo dyes, non-azo dyes, and preservatives in a population of perennial asthmatics. *J Allergy Clin Immunol* 1979;64:32–37.
207. Weinberg IG, Tuchinda M: Allergic tension-fatigue syndrome. *Ann Allergy* 1973;31:209–211.
208. Weiss TJ: *Food Oils.* Westport, CT, Avi Publishing Co, 1970.
209. Wergeland J: Three fatal cases of probable familial allergy to human milk. *Acta Paed* 1948;35:321–334.
210. White PL: The lid is off. *JAMA* 1981;238:1761–1762.
211. Whitehead SB, Shaw FR: *Honeybees and Their Management.* New York, D. Van Nostrand Co, 1951, p 148.
212. Wicher K, Reisman RE, Arbesman CE: Allergic reaction to penicillin in milk. *JAMA* 1969;208:143–145.
213. Wilson E: Preventive medicine as illustrated in the proper use of food. *Am J Med Sc* 1865;49:534–539.
214. Wilson JF, Lahey ME, Heiner DC: Studies on iron metabolism. V. Further observations on cow's milk-induced bleeding in infants with iron-deficiency anemia. *J Pediatr* 1974;84:335–344.
215. Wolf SI: Tension-fatigue syndrome. *Clin Proc Children's Hosp* 1971;27:25–35.

216. Wolff IA, Wasserman AE: Nitrates, nitrites and nitrosamines. *Science* 1972;177:15–18.
217. Wooton WT: Allergy: an everyday problem. *J Arkansas Med Ass* 1934; 31:71–74.
218. Wright R, Truelove SC: Trial of various diets in ulcerative colitis. *Br Med J* 1965;2:138.
219. Ziegler WH: *The Meat We Eat.* Danville, IL, Interstate Printers & Publishers, 1948, ed 5, pp 326–331.
220. Ziering WH: Otitis media and milk allergy (letter). *Pediatrics* 1973;51: 154–155.

INDEX

Besides this index, consult also the following alphabetical listings: for individual plant foods and plant-food families, Chapter 4, pp 39–67; for plant and animal foods, Chapter 5, pp 69–152, and Chapter 8, pp 171–196.